How Life Moves

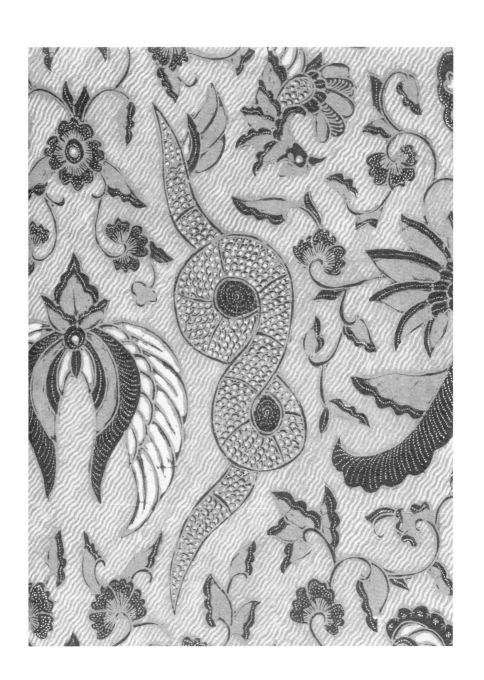

How Life Moves

EXPLORATIONS IN
MEANING AND BODY AWARENESS

Caryn McHose
and
Kevin Frank

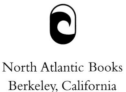

North Atlantic Books
Berkeley, California

Published by North Atlantic Books
P.O. Box 12327, Berkeley, California 94712

Cover photo by Kevin Frank
Cover design by Susan Kress Hamilton
Book design by Susan Kress Hamilton
Frontispiece: "Snake" (detail of Indonesian textile)

Printed in the United States of America

How Life Moves, Explorations in Meaning and Body Awareness is sponsored by the Society for the Study of Native Arts and Sciences, a nonprofit educational corporation whose goals are to develop an educational and crosscultural perspective linking various scientific, social, and artistic fields; to nurture a holistic view of arts, sciences, humanities, and healing; and to publish and distribute literature on the relationship of mind, body, and nature.

North Atlantic Books' publications are available through most bookstores. For further information, call 800-337-2665 or visit our website at www.northatlanticbooks.com.

Substantial discounts on bulk quantities are available to corporations, professional associations, and other organizations. For details and discount information, contact our special sales department.

ISBN 978-1-55643-618-5

Library of Congress Cataloging-in-Publication Data

McHose, Caryn, 1952-
  How life moves : explorations in meaning and body awareness / by Caryn
McHose and Kevin Frank.
       p. cm.
    Summary: "An experiential movement curriculum with a cutting edge approach
to perception and body awareness—an in-depth manual for body workers, yoga
practitioners, movement teachers, dancers, physical, somatic, and
psychological therapists, theater students, and for anyone wanting to
understand the principles beneath posture, movement, and body/mind
training"—Provided by publisher.
  Includes bibliographical references and index.
  ISBN 1-55643-618-1
  1. Movement education. I. Frank, Kevin, 1951– II. Society for the Study
of Native Arts and Sciences. III. Title.
  GV452.M37 2006
  372.86'8—dc22
                                          2006001935

2 3 4 5 6 7 8 9 United 12 11 10 09 08 07

Contents

Acknowledgments

We honor colleagues and teachers who helped us in our exploration of imagery, sensation, and perception in movement. The body of ideas and the experiences they offer are so significant we have provided an appendix to summarize some of their work. Here we would like to thank those with whom we have studied, and continue to study, for their contributions to our work.

Thank you to the Rolf Institute® and, by extension, to Ida P. Rolf for her theory and practice of structural integration.

Thanks to Hubert Godard for the theory of tonic function and a continuing exploration of its application. We particularly thank him for all the time and effort he has devoted to working with us.

Thanks to Susan Harper for her work in imagery, sensation, and emotion; to Emilie Conrad, whose brilliant work is all about liberation from habit; to Toni Packer, who tirelessly encourages to notice this moment; and to Bonnie Bainbridge Cohen for her inspiration to consider the body systems, as well as developmental and evolutionary patterns.

Thank you to Peter Levine for revolutionizing the treatment of shock and trauma, and for providing a model of self-empowerment through somatic awareness.

We would like to acknowledge Betty Jane Dittmar, an innovative teacher of dance. Betty Jane recognizes the inherent creativity that every person has and empowers all to access their unique capacity to find this for themselves through movement.

We thank Susan Borg for her inquiry and innovation in sound and movement education and for the many years of teaching and exploring together. We thank Andrea Olsen for holding the space of creativity and spirit in dance and art, and for continued collaboration. We thank Tom Myers, who helped clarify our perceptions of structure and evolution.

For somatic education in many forms, we thank Ticia Agri, James Asher, Rosemary Feitis, Hans Flury, Eric Hawkins, James Jealous, Deane Juhan, Arthur Kilmurray, Jeffrey Maitland, Ray McCall, Michael Murphy, Aline Newton, Konrad Obermeier, Gael Ohlgren, James Oschman, Michael Salveson, Louis Schultz, Robert Shleip, Tom Shaver, William Smythe, Jan Sultan, Charles Swenson, and Ron Thompson.

For teaching with the knowledge that creativity dwells within each of us, we thank Cynthia Snow.

For holding space, we thank Carole Burstein, Linda Westfall, Paula France, Candace Loubert, and Martha Whitney.

For design, artwork, and creative vision, we thank Susan Kress Hamilton.

For photography, we thank John Hession, who met the challenge in many ways.

Other photos are by Peggy Keon, Jay O'Rear, Carol Zickel, and Carlo Chiulli. For art consultation, we thank Deborah Wilding. We thank Galen Beach for drawings and other artwork. Thank you to Critters in Crisis Movement Studio.

We thank Serge Gracovetsky for images from *The Spinal Engine*. We thank John Wexo for illustrations from *Prehistoric Zoobooks*. We thank Vicki Pearse for illustrations from *Animals without Backbones*. We thank Chris Newbert and Brigitte Wilms for their underwater photos.

For support and editorial genius, we thank Liz Wilding.

For movement participation, we thank Susan Borg, Brittany Cobb, Chadwick Cobb, Chantilly Cobb, Chesterton Cobb, Richard Nesson, Kyle Nicholas, Courtney Schmidt, Savannah Swan, Audrey Swift, Deborah Wilding, and Liz Wilding.

We thank other movement participants: Brooks Whitehouse, Janet Ornstein, Gene Podhurst, Claire Arneson, Sandy MacNeill, Carol Zickell, Siana Goodwin, Theresa Zink, Stell Snyder, Gordon Snyder, Linnea Snyder, Vernonique Mead, Malcolm Manning, Colleen Bartley, Sophia Diamantopoulou, Susan Hayes, Susanna Recchia, Andrea Olsen, Karen Smith, Margaret Ames, and Adele Levi.

We thank the George and Ann Levin for the use of their beach. We thank Eugenia West, and Bob and Lili Young for the use of their fields.

Thanks to Eeva-Maria Mutka and Andy Paget for creating a space that holds this work.

For life lessons and early support, we thank Joy and Andre McHose, and Tim and Hally Sheely.

We thank our students and clients, with whom we explore the frontiers of perception and movement. We acknowledge teachers who take the risk of proposing that people explore movement. We also acknowledge the mystery of life, and its infinite creativity in movement.

We dedicate this book to Lawrence K. Frank, 1890–1968, a founder of the child development movement who argued that the central problem of child development research was to understand the development of the whole child and who advocated that research be child-centered by understanding that children are emerging, becoming, and dynamically learning.

Caryn McHose and Kevin Frank
Holderness, New Hampshire

HUBERT GODARD

Foreword
Translated from the French

This book is an adventure, a risk. The authors venture into the thousand facets that comprise the appearance of an action.

This book invites the reader to inhabit a place without words, where the roots of habitual movement live, pre-conscious and unknown. It is a sensitive and vulnerable journey in movement.

It involves sharing and describing body movement as it is, experienced by each individual, without betraying the precious history of events that have formed our lives and shaped our vocabulary of movement. This promotes a new perspective, at the edge of our usual ways of doing and feeling.

This process arouses difficult questions shared by all therapists, movement instructors, and teachers of dance, yoga, martial arts, and sports.

The stumbling blocks are great. Professionals often project the way they experience movement, their own stories, upon their students. This may, of course, encourage a sense of openness in the students, but it may also cause them to adopt an artificial framework that will muddle their sense of spontaneity, which is necessary for any fluid expression. This could also result in the imposition of a mechanistic vision that corresponds to an anatomical truth or an error in teaching because each individual's specific characteristics

are not taken into account. Indeed, there is a long list of pitfalls.

The authors' bias delights us. Insofar as no formulaic lesson has been given, respect and attention are lavished here upon each person's specific process. This type of know-how is not invented. It is forged in the silence of studios and the many years of experimentation with movement and how it is taught.

There is simplicity here, and we detect erudition regarding the body, which is essential to the multi-disciplinary knowledge needed to analyze and teach body movement. This authorship is a fortunate meeting of two unique life paths. This meeting combines areas as disparate as comparative anatomy, functional anatomy, phylogenesis, psychology, clinical orthopedics, dance, and somatic techniques. Knowledge regarding the teaching of movement does not constitute a discipline in itself, so every researcher in this area needs to build an eclectic body of knowledge. The authors never obstruct the simple, yet deep, proposals that guide the creation of body movements that can astonish us, that direct us toward unknown lands, a potential that we have not contemplated.

Caryn McHose and Kevin Frank lead us to an investigation that uses phylogenic development, from the first original cell to the animals that we

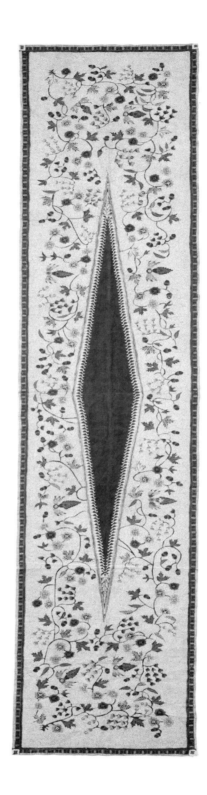

are today, as its metaphor. This journey through organic time guides us toward an examination of the way in which we perceive our bodies in motion in relation to the world.

The details of proprioceptive information, the feeling of a flesh-and-blood self that is dealing with its context, is the keystone that lends meaning to the emergence of body movement and, consequently, to the establishment of an identity. It is here that we measure the fragility of any educational action. The awareness of the options we chose in the twists and turns of emerging sensation involve not only the material progression of body movement, but also, in the background, our position with regard to others and the security of a constant self, despite the fact that the next body movement is still unknown.

This security, this need for constancy, is articulated around one single permanent event that provides us with the context: the force of earthly gravity. In living beings, this force leads to a second force that is unique to each individual. Each movement comes about through a force that opposes gravity. This game, this dialogue, this struggle, or this cooperation will serve as the raw material for the gesture.

The hazards of our relationship to gravity and its variations in tone are fraught with history. This is the only information that a newborn perceives with regard to those who are around him or her. Gravity is the organizational movement beneath his or her first dialogues and interpersonal exchanges. The newborn does not yet have the power of symbolic construction or language to back and support a particular meaning. He or she only perceives variations in tone, rhythm, and melody in others, as well as accentuations and intensities that are reflected by faces and bodies. He or she will respond in kind. This creates a field of exchanges and meanings that are later used as the framework for the development of language, symbols, and movements.

"Genesis of Space" (Indonesian textile).
(Photograph by John Hession.)

The vertical axis of gravity will be used to shoulder and support everything that comprises our visceral, respiratory, circulatory, and motor functions, all of which are major phenomena that shape the way in which we stand up to the world.

Our relationship with weight and spatial orientation is never self-evident because it is overlaid with all the events that constituted our first relationships. We can only perceive an objective "weight-related self" through the veil of subjectivity, through the meaning that each individual gives to his or her affective history.

The images, metaphors, and movements in this book encourage the exploration of how we move and feel in our real life. They help us travel the path from present-time context to the moments of early life when we intertwined gravity with our relational dilemma. The proprioceptive act, as the knowledge and consciousness of our own movements in gravity, spills over onto all perception-related phenomena. The act of perception, whatever it may be, is not separable from the intention to explore and not separable from the object that is being sensed. What my hand feels depends on palpatory muscular activity and the internal map of my body, as well as on my preconception of the object that I have touched.

By the same token, the way we look at things depends on the activity of our eye muscles, which are, in turn, subjected to the direction of gravity by the mechanisms of the inner ear and the meaning that our affective signature assigns to the various objects that we observe.

The four structures described here—our physical structure, the structure of our coordinations (the orchestration of both muscular and sensory work), the structure of our perceptive habits, and the structure of our psychic composition—all control the work of our imagination.

As many authors have emphasized, the work of our imagination and our perception both refer to one single phenomenon. The teacher's function should be to rehabilitate the imagination in areas of fixation.

The proposals set forth here are intended for all of our senses, because they must all function in harmony. We now know the extent to which each sensory channel is influenced by the activity of other channels, and often the only way to go beyond a limit on perception will be to fuel it first through the use of another sense.

Using awareness to guide an experience related to body movement and associating this movement with tactile, sound, olfactory, or kinesthetic information often allows us to get past trouble spots.

We must have a generous amount of educational knowledge reflecting a willingness to listen to others, to be able to detect each person's own form of logic. Often, failings with regard to our imagination are linked to the activity of one single sensory mode. The ability to navigate through the diverse range of felt senses offers the gesture traveler the joy of discovering new territory.

It is essential to point out that the space in which we carry out our movement is not homogenous. It is eminently subjective, composed of various densities linked to the history of the types of happiness and sadness that we have experienced. It is populated by the ghostly traces of our past encounters and the meaning that we will have assigned to these events.

Our presence in the location that surrounds us will be accomplished irregularly, for example, more to the right or to the left, more toward the bottom than toward the top, more toward the back than the front, and so on. The same can be said for the comfort distance that we maintain with regard to others; this distance is unique to each person. In the same way, we have a unique visual perspective when we observe our surroundings.

A car accident may sometimes leave us closed off, subconsciously fearing the direction in which the collision took place. Thus neglected, the points that dot the space need to be conquered again and repopulated, so that we can reopen our potential for action in these directions. The distortions of our physical structure often reflect the perils of this imaginary construction of space, and one of this book's strong points is its ability to tackle this question delicately and relevantly. Manuals that discuss techniques of movement often limit their focus to how the body notices itself rather than how the body notices the space surrounding it.

This "gravity-related me," the line of force that built our relationship to weight and our sense of vertical line, as well as the variations of our subjective space, all define the limits of our bodies and our boundaries with regard to others. The ease with which we project ourselves, express ourselves in society, and the facility with which we receive the presence of others form an adaptive boundary that should be responsive to any given situation.

Today's lifestyles have brought about a considerable degree of relational fragility, and demands for the resolution of these difficulties are loud and clear. There are many current proposals to help people strengthen their ability to feel at ease in social situations. The path proposed here is not reduced to behavioral response (typically composed of partial formulas concerning the way to communicate, express, and receive). The authors have adopted a radical stance. They ask us to consider the origin of that which creates the "expressive, social me." In each of the chapters, various fundamental aspects of this question are tackled in a playful, exploratory spirit that helps overcome the fears associated with this area.

The authors focus on the more general question of our repertory, our potential for gesture, as well as our inhibited body movements, whether absent or repressed. Here, the work is about going back to the beginning, toward basic root body movements that can serve as points of departure for a more complex look at our repertory. Foundational gestures, such as reaching toward, pushing back, pointing, cutting, and so on, are explored at their origins. Movement begins with the selection of sensory information and its specific relationship to gravity and space. Difficulties linked to execution or inhibitions will be overcome only at these levels of investigation.

The alternation of free and guided movements, the meaning given to what supports us, to group experiences, to interactions with others, to the body movement's points of spatial and bodily initiation, to the image of our moving body, of our welcoming space, will help to restart and enrich imaginary function. In this eleven-chapter voyage, four approaches are used:

• The first approach comprises knowledge that provides a basis for exploration and offers an entry that helps build the context of experience. This knowledge is essential to deconstruct the culture beneath our mind set. The reason I say "culture" is that these conceptual sets would be very different if we lived in China, for example, even though we are still concerned with the same human body that obeys the same organic laws. All of these cultural data and beliefs shape our perceptions, our coordinations, and their resultant gestures, often without our knowledge. The language that we use influences our perception. A language designs a specific body that is preconceived, pre-perceived, in accordance with the linguistic potential offered by that particular language.

• The second approach is the opposite of the first and, in fact, involves the telling of personal stories, gleaned by the authors during their teaching. This approach enables us to penetrate the more subjective, emotional dimension of movement as it is experienced and perceived according to the uniqueness that is exclusive to each individual. These very moving accounts let us grasp and imagine a set of phenomena that cognitive approach cannot cover. Through direct empathy, the student discovers what others have experienced and may then make associations with his or her own experiences.

• The third approach involves the description of a movement problem that follows from the first two approaches. At this point we are inside the realm of "doing" and of the act of creation. After concept and affect, we enter the world of percept. Our imagination, prepared by other approaches, will deal with motor situations, either known or unknown, and this approach moves past the limits of how we usually do and feel things. The major question with regard to gesture, as we know it, rests on how sharply and efficiently we grasp information about the world and about ourselves. The clarity of the explorations proposed here will help us.

• Finally, the last approach, intended for teachers and therapists, tries to unveil educational strategies, the why and the how of the exercises that have proved effective in the authors' wide experience. It goes without saying that this is intended for every individual, regardless of whether he or she is a teacher, to the extent that we are our own first teachers, especially in the field of gesture.

All these propositions can be seen as an odyssey. Like Ulysses' return to his native island, the body movement that belongs exclusively to each of us must be invented through a thousand ruses in order to deal with the obstacles and mirages that separate us from our goal. But this also extends to the comparison with Penelope, who did not hesitate to untie her weaving every day. We must undo our perceptions and coordinations daily to extend the moment of possibility, and allow again the new gesture to come.

Introduction

This book is experiential in nature. It is about movement and the exploration of perception, imagination, and sensation. We present a theoretical base, exercises, and imagery that can support liberation from habituated patterns of movement and the opportunity to move in more healthy ways.

This book sets out to meet two goals. The first goal is to outline a versatile context for teaching people about perception and body shape, as they relate to structure and function. The second goal is to ask questions about the learning process itself: What supports us in learning to shift our body shape, our movement, and our relationships?

There is interplay between perception, imagination, and sensation both in habituated movement and creative, healing movement.

All of us have habituated patterns of movement that help us respond to our environment efficiently, even instantly. Our habitual movements are based on our perceptions. Perception can be defined as the way each of us organizes the stream of sensory information that arises in any moment.

We respond to what we perceive. But what do we perceive? Is our interpretation of the world, our sensation of the world, real or imagined—or a blend of the two?

We learn to perceive in a series of encounters with the world involving all of the senses. Our

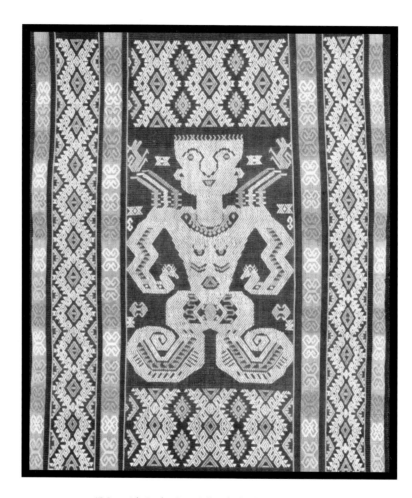

"Man with Snake Arms" (detail of Indonesian textile).

learning is affected by culture, family, and personal experience. We learn to think of ourselves as having gender, size, and human shape. We move the way we see others move and the way that "feels" comfortable, emotionally as well as in sensation.

We have within us images of the world, images of ourselves, and images of movements that we depend on to navigate the world. What we perceive and how we move is mostly confined to the closet of these images.

Our bodies also have a capacity to locate where they are in any moment. Our ability to sense location in gravity is called proprioception. Proprioception is not confined to memory and image.

When our interpretation of sensation is based on memory and past experience, the body-mind "makes up" the perception it experiences. This is interesting territory for the student of movement. What if, some of the time, we interrupt our routines of perception? Is it possible to perceive something free of our past habits? Is it possible to use imagination in a way that liberates our perception and movement? Can we form new perceptions?

In this book we introduce a set of exercises based on our experience with changing perception. We can learn to orient to sensation and use imagery to notice sensations freshly, if we use imagery that speaks to proprioception. From that fresh noticing of sensation, our perceptions of the world or our body, and even our beliefs can be unlocked from habit. Then, rather than create a new belief or idea, we can continue to notice sensation in the present moment. We can begin to observe the difference between perception from habit and perception that is new.

I may temporarily shift body image or map of my environment because I pause to notice what is sensate, what is new and alive in this moment. When I go to move again, the preparation to move is based on fresh information. Now it is possible to have an innovated movement.

From nature and evolution, we have found imagery that provides organizing metaphors for our exercises. These metaphors can foster new perception. In particular we use the metaphor of the evolutionary story. We use our experience of weight, space, and directionality to inform the body as we explore metaphor. Noticing the present moment through our senses is also a part of finding new perception.

What happens when we stop thinking of ourselves as only human and explore, through imagination, our similarities to other creatures that have evolved with us? How might creatures experience space and weight—how do they move? And how can we move as them, as them within us? Is there an experience of resonance with these creatures that can help us to find new movements?

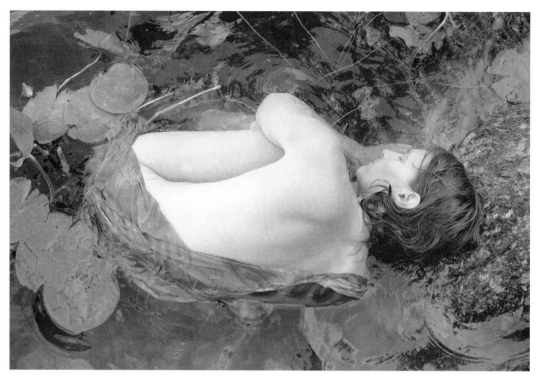

Photograph by Carlo Chiulli.

An Inquiry into Movement Education— Perception, Movement, Structure, Metaphor, and Imagination

PERCEPTION

Our world exists because we sense it, interpret it, and build a perception. We sense our body and we sense our environment. From these sensations we build a map of our internal and external world. If we are open and curious, as we are in infancy, sensations stimulate us—they grab our attention. Once we are stimulated by sensations, we are awakened to new perception and this leads to new body shape, and movement impulse.

The senses are our doorway to perception. Sensations are to-whom-it-may-concern messages from our skin, our sense organs, our muscles and organs, to our brain. Most of these messages arrive unnoticed. The noticed ones constitute perception. Perception is the interpretation we make of our sensation.

Learning to move is an experiment in interaction. No movement springs fully formed. Nor does our environment imprint movement upon us. We try things out, tentatively, awkwardly, sometimes directly and easily. We learn to do what is successful. This, in turn, becomes automatic.

Movement is also the result of the culture and particular family into which we are born. We perceive others in our environment and strive to move in similar ways.

At the outset, learning to move starts with a flow of sensations and the development of perception. How one perceives oneself and the environment will shape the impulse to experiment.

My perception and sensation are intricately bound. Sound, color, or smell, any of these, will stimulate a cascade of feeling—feeling for which my infant body had no name. From raw, unstructured feeling, I rapidly develop perception, a way of knowing and recognizing the pattern of feeling. Each perception will develop an accompanying meaning.

If I smell something and I am not very sensitive to scent, the sensation of smell may arouse me only a little and I may only slightly orient to the scent. If scent makes a big impression, or if my caretakers express excitement when there is a new scent, then smell becomes a more powerful focus in my perception. I may lean forward. I may lift my head to capture the new scent. The shape and direction of my movement, the posture I adopt, will reflect the story of my perception.

LANGUAGE

Language affects perception. Observe how language shapes what you see, hear, taste, and feel. Language styles profoundly affect our picture of the world. This book introduces words that may be unfamiliar or have a strong association. Since words can have a big effect, we will give you opportunity to slow down and notice their effect on you.

MOVEMENT, HABITUATION, AND CHANGE

School-age children and most adults are typically captives in a world that discourages experimentation and curiosity. Most of us are taught to avoid risk in learning and to find answers quickly. In most learning contexts, it is the goal rather than the process that is valued.

It is also true that learning to move has urgency for any creature. Birds, deer, and mosquitoes all need to learn their movements quickly so they are more likely to survive.

In humans, goal orientation and urgency to survive lead to habits of inhibition that get in the way of learning new and better movement. These habits are hard to change. The result is that many people, especially those living in modern cultures, are losing their capacity for healthy, effective movement. Inhibition, along with a life in chairs, cars, and couches, leads to obesity and a variety of musculoskeletal problems.

It is possible to learn new movement now—at any stage of life—movement that can help to support health and healing. This learning is actually mostly "unlearning." Unlearning is a challenge, especially when it is about unlearning things that were learned with a sense of survival at stake. Unlearning is possible. It happens at the level of perception. Unlearning happens in the preparation to move. That preparation is mutable at the bridge between sensation and meaning. This bridge is perception.

For example, low back pain is a common problem, a result of the lost capacity to move in healthy, fluid concert with our musculoskeletal system.

Low back pain can involve muscle contractions that conflict with each other, that overtighten our joints and squeeze nerves. Reorganization of perception, based on imagery and a return to sensation, can enable those core muscles to work in fluid coordination again.

The evolutionary story provides possibilities for shifting movements that underlie the maladies of modern life, such as low back, shoulder, or neck pain.

Many systems of movement and bodywork address such maladies. Our own training derives partly from the work of Ida Rolf and more specifically of Hubert Godard. *(See Appendix A for a more complete discussion of their work and influence.)*

Rolf developed structural integration, a way of using fascial reorganization to produce equilibrium in the body.

Godard adds to structural integration his theory of tonic function. Tonic function is a model that describes orientation and the body's preparation for movement. How we orient to weight and space, how our body prepares to move while orienting, and how we shift perception to change our pre-movement—these are key factors in making lasting improvements in back pain and all musculoskeletal complaints. Orientation through a sense of weight in the body and orientation to space enable us to restore healthy movement.

FOUR STRUCTURES OF MOVEMENT AND THEIR RELATIONSHIP TO CHANGE

In our approach to movement learning, we consider four kinds of structure: physical, perceptual, coordinative, and meaning.[1]

In this book we primarily focus on the last three.[2] That is because physical structure is affected by shifts in any of the other three structures and ultimately will be the long-term measure of our success.[3]

Tonic function theory also says that by using these four structures as parameters, we can observe and describe many of the dimensions that predict movement. Our survival depends on predictability in movement. Structure allows this. Skill in considering these dimensions of structure can help us support healthy innovation in movement. We find that the development of skillful observation begins in the senses.

If we wish to change human movement, we must be clever enough to stimulate change in structures that aren't designed to be changed casually. If a movement strategy was very mutable, what good would it be when your life depended on it? Adaptability in movement is good, but random and easily shifted structure would quickly lead to accidents and misfortune, as those living with chronic neurological disease or easily dislocated joints can attest. How can we benevolently affect movement structure? What *is* movement structure?

PHYSICAL STRUCTURE

Physical structure encompasses the physical elements of the body that change slowly over time. This includes the size and shape of bone, muscle, fascia, organs, nerves, and so on. Your physical structure is partly the result of genetics. It is also the product of your environment, and the ways you have learned to perceive, coordinate, and make meaning. In other words, physical structure derives from the other three structures. That is why it is so important to consider these other structures if we wish to make lasting changes in musculoskeletal health.

We might describe physical structure as follows. If you stand upright, your postural shape describes a particular "structure" that in unguarded moments will be quite predictable. Your feet will face in certain directions; your knees will be flexed, extended, or rotated; your hips will slant in different ways—all the way up to your head.

If we examine the texture and tone of the soft tissue, we could begin to map the way that soft tissue helps you assume a fairly consistent shape. Similarly, we can map the angles and positions of all the bones. Physical structure is what most body therapists mean when they talk about structure.

PERCEPTUAL STRUCTURE

Perceptual structures are less easy to differentiate. If asked to report what you are sensing, your report will reflect your habits of perception. You might, for example, immediately report that you are hearing distant sounds. That in turn might lead you to notice sensations in your neck and shoulders. We could map your tendency, your habits of perception, by listening to your reports, or by watching you carefully. This would start to describe your perceptual structure.

Perceptual structure helps us organize the stream of sensate messages so that life is efficient. We don't have to invent our body response over and over again, to manage incoming sensations.

However, the perception that we create is just that—a creation. It is a creation of our mind, selective reconstruction of the actual world.

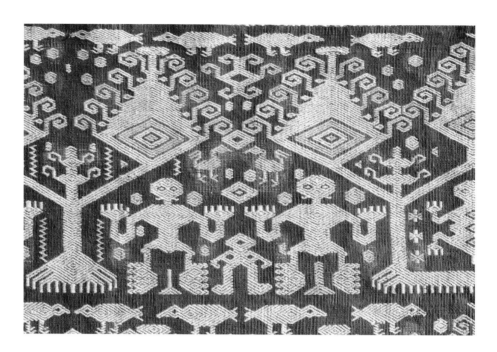

Fig. 1.2. *"Humans" (detail of Indonesian textile).*

Perhaps you can already sense the potency and value of perceptual change.

COORDINATIVE STRUCTURE

Coordinative structure is another fundamental building block of movement. In coordinative structure we look at the way the body creates movement subroutines. We call on these subroutines for most of our common tasks without repeatedly having to invent them. Each of these subroutines is composed of combinations of muscle recruitment the body knows will work.

You express a coordinative structure when you tie your shoes. To tie shoes you use a certain learned sequence of moves in the dance of your fingers and laces. If a close friend or relative watches a video of your hands tying your shoes, she will quickly recognize the movement as belonging to you. The movement pattern is like a fingerprint, unique to you. Also, notice that after the first fifty times, you don't really have to think about doing this task. After enough rehearsal, the complexity of tying your shoes doesn't take a lot of brainpower. That's because subroutines now engage automatically.

MEANING STRUCTURE

Meaning structure is the story that helps you keep track of your perceptions, especially with regard to perceptions about your self and your environment—that is, self and other. Meaning keeps perceptions associated with stories so you know what to do in response to those perceptions, and that may immediately trigger the beginning of the next movement.

You have meaning structures that affect your movement and your posture. If you enter a library, or a forest, or a church, each place will affect you. Your posture and movements will shift in subtle or obvious ways. They are associated with the story of what these places have meant to you in your life. Each place will touch the meaning-making part of you. Conversely, assuming a certain posture can evoke the meaning story associated with that shape of your body. For example, genuflection may evoke church. Usually these meanings are predictable and habitual. But again, as meaning changes, movement can begin to change.

Discovering new body perceptions is a powerful way to shift the quality of a person's movement and improve function. Attending to sensations, dwelling in pre-reflective, story-free episodes of awareness can liberate movement from function—function being movement with a goal attached to it. Moving and attending in a mood of simple curiosity allows the body's habits to release. This work, if it is going to shift or change quality of movement, has to be about unlocking habits—of movement, perception, coordination, and meaning-making.

All these structures are tendencies that will predict what will occur as a person prepares to move. In this book we offer innovative exercises that can shift the three structures underlying movement: perceptual, coordinative, and meaning.

THE USE OF METAPHOR AND STORY TO SUPPORT STRUCTURAL CHANGE

Metaphor can help to inform perception, coordination, and meaning. By metaphor we mean the use of an image or idea to help understand something analogous. It is an effective way of communicating with people and is complementary to the direct manipulation found in many types of bodywork.

Stories are made up of metaphors. We are all familiar with the use of parables and folk tales that inform the way we live. Each person or animal symbolizes some element of our experience. We all have stories for the way we move and the movements themselves are built of metaphors derived from our past experience.

Telling stories is the oldest form of passing on knowledge and invoking the imagination. As soon as I tell you a story about my history, or the history of something you are interested in, you make pictures in your mind. Those pictures inform you about some aspect of life. The pictures are your metaphors for what I tell you. You become active in your imagination. Imagination can then be used to discover new sensations, perceptions, and possibly new movement.

Some stories are easier to relate to than others. The trick may be to find the safe and available starting point for each person. It's hard to teach something new without referring to some story of your past, although it is possible. Story and metaphor are powerful tools for teaching movement and for helping shift structure.

The evolutionary story is the metaphor for the exercises in this book. Science has compared the present life forms with those in fossil records, and has constructed a story about adaptation and progression. Within the evolutionary story are creatures that share many biological characteristics with us. Those creatures can be used as metaphors for our own exploration of sensation and movement. Evolution and nature are doorways to perception. The evolutionary story affects us because it refers to biology that is a part of who and what we are. The shapes of the different kinds of animals, from one-celled creatures to complex mammals, all speak to us, touch us, because they are familiar. We have single cells within us, as well as many of the functions and shapes of the creatures that preceded us or developed in tandem with our own evolution.

For example, the hydra is a present-day animal whose body is a metaphor for our human digestive system. After all, that is what a hydra is—a digestive system in the form of a hollow tube that plants itself on the bottom of a lake. We have within us the potential to feel a hydra-like part of us. Seeing a picture of a hydra, and then imagining what it would feel like to be one, we can have a sensory experience that makes the hydra less abstract. This makes our digestive system more interesting to feel, and can lead to startlingly different ways of moving.

As I begin to move my body in slow, quiet resonance with the hydra, I find new ways to move. The perception of flow and space in the hydra enable me to relearn how to move, to heal and to adapt.

The creature stories, the movements I imagine, can be metaphors for my own movement. This is about exploration and imagination rather than literal translation.

Ontogeny does not repeat phylogeny. Human embryological development does not mirror biological evolution. That debate has been laid to rest. However, the history of life forms on the planet is a history of anatomical change coupled with attempts to survive and reproduce, to adapt to the environment. Anatomical changes changed movement. Changes in environment challenged creatures to adapt. We see a similar story when we observe the growth of the human being from infancy to adulthood. Movement class provides an opportunity for experimentation with, and adaptation to, new contexts and movement challenges.

The evolutionary story offers us biological forms interacting with their environment and sets a context for broad exploration with movement, perception, and meaning.

MOVEMENT EDUCATION

As students in, and teachers of, movement classes, all of us can make important shifts in how we move in the world. We offer some suggestions about what works, and why, and then give you the opportunity to find out how you learn.

Movement study occurs best through inquiry. We define inquiry as a two-step process that involves asking the question "What is true for me in this moment?" And then the question "What else could be true for me in this moment?" In particular, we are asking these questions as they pertain to experimentation in imagination, sensation, perception, coordination, and movement. We are inviting you to let your body experience be your most important teacher.

We claim from the outset that "new" movement possibilities, freedom from restriction, and the joy of creativity in our movements of thought, body, and feeling (body, feeling, and thought?) are the province of the natural animal body if it can be liberated from the confines of human habit.

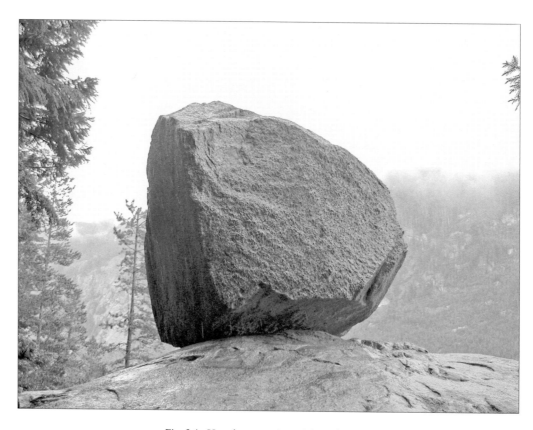

Fig. 2.1. *How do we perceive weight and space?*

CHAPTER 2

Orientation –
Child of Heaven and Earth

As you begin your journey into the various realms of animal body, first stop at an earlier and more basic moment of creation.

Before there is an animal body or any body at all, there is the polarity of weight and space.[1] The universe is a place of mass. Mass bestows weight. The universe is also mostly space. The universe is a place of condensation and pressure, and a place of expansion and vastness.

As small beings in the universe, we have mass. We have weight. We are simultaneously a piece of the universe that is mostly space, so we are also space. This is not something we typically notice and allow to touch our awareness. What is your association to the terms *weight* and *space*? What is your body's response?

Which interests you most, weight or space? What is the felt sense that arises? By felt sense we mean a sensory feeling that emerges as our overall body sense for any particular moment. Move, draw, or make a sound that expresses the felt sense of weight or space.

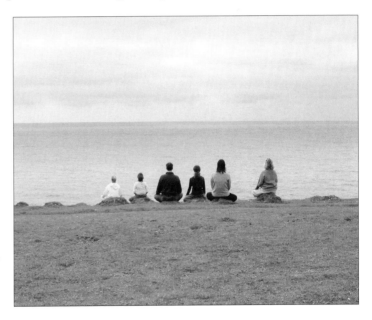

Fig. 2.2. *Orientation.*

What happens for you? Here are some reports by students we have worked with:

"As soon as you said **space***, I felt calm and noticed I was less worried about the time and how long we were going to be here. I felt a smoothing sensation in my chest and belly. I drew a picture of colored spirals emerging from a hub."*

"I didn't like thinking about the term **weight** *but I was more drawn to thinking about it anyway. I notice sensations of irritability. I guess that's an emotion. The sensation is burning/itching in my calves and belly and throat. Then I moved and I jumped up and down until there was a sensation of heaviness. That felt pleasant."*

All of us, who have grown up on a planet and lived on land, are children of both weight and space. Our biology is linked to the sense of weight and space *(Fig. 2.3)*. We call this link to weight and space *gravity orientation*. The system within us that performs this orientation is our gravity response system.

Gravity orientation is the substructure upon which the other four structures (physical, perceptual, coordinative, and meaning) are built. Orientation makes it possible for perception to have a perceiver. By learning about gravity, we are empowered to make dramatic shifts in the structures underlying our movement patterns and our relational life. We have weight and space. Each of us organizes around weight and space differently, and this affects the way we move in relation to others.

The way to learn about gravity orientation starts by finding some ways of intentionally shifting it. Then we can start to notice that we are always held by both aspects of gravity. We are held between heaven and earth.

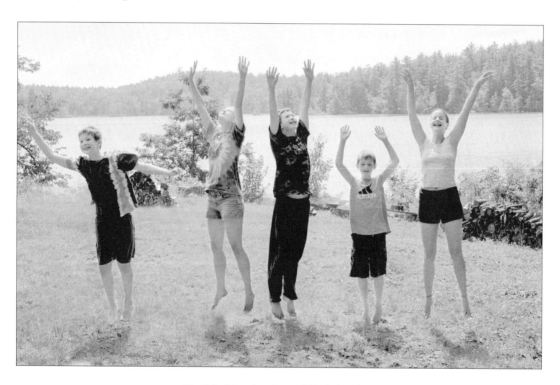

Fig. 2.3. *Moon jumping and Earth jumping.*

Here are three exercises that are helpful in feeling the two sides of gravity. The first is a group exercise.

Group Exercise:
LIMBS RADIATING FROM THE CENTER

Divide your group in two. One half of the group starts jumping up and down, then pauses and starts jumping up and down again. The other half watches. See if you can notice the Earth jumpers and the Moon jumpers. Earth jumpers go down to go up. They start by amplifying their weight and mass primarily in the legs and feet. Moon jumpers start with a sense of excitement about the space into which they can launch. After you jumped without thinking about it, see if you can try the other option. How do the two options feel? Do you find any experience of weight or mass? Do you notice what it means to amplify a sense of space? Is one way of jumping harder or easier?

Exercise:
EARTH BODY/SKY BODY

Another exercise can be done outside or simply in the imagination. Can you remember a time when you lay on the ground and either joined the Earth in its movement or the sky and the clouds in their movement? Can you feel the sense of weight that lets you feel that you are the Earth? Can you feel yourself as Earth turning and allow the clouds to pass by? Can you, by contrast, stare up at the clouds and be with the sense of space and clouds? Can you feel yourself as clouds floating, drifting, and expanding? Then, can you notice your Earth aspect and sky-cloud aspect at the same time? Which aspect is easier to feel? *(See Fig. 2.4).*

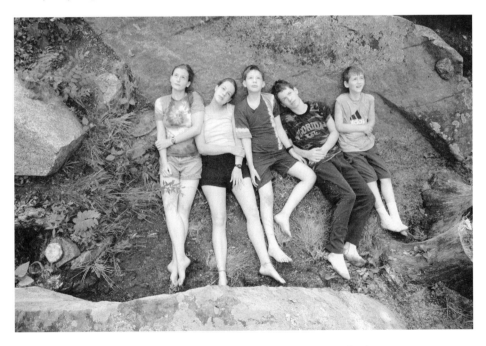

Fig. 2.4. *Children accepting the invitation to notice the sky.*

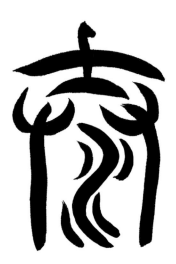

Fig. 2.5. *Chinese character representing T'ai, the 11th hexagram of the I Ching, Heaven and Earth: "Two essences that harmoniously merge are an expression of T'ai."*[2] (Drawing by Galen Beach.)

Exercise:
Space Inside/Space Outside

Press your hands together. Rub them vigorously against each other, back and forth. After your hands get hot, stop and see what you notice. What do you notice in sensation, specifically? If your sensation includes movement, is it inside your hands or between them? If you feel the inside, can you feel the between? Is the reverse possible? Can you go back and forth?

You have just exercised a shift between weight and space orientation. The inside-the-hands feeling will count in this example as weight orientation. The between-the-hands feeling is an orientation to space.

Are there other possibilities? Yes, there are. In this instance if you noticed a different possibility, see if you can make a connection to the inside-versus-outside contrast.

GRAVITY ORIENTATION AND PERCEPTION

In the same way that you shifted your sense of substance or movement from inside the hands to between the hands, we can shift any of our senses from weight orientation to space orientation. We can look out at the world or we can feel the world touch our eyes. We can hear the sounds far away or we can allow the sounds to touch our ears and bones. We will find that these two different ways of perceiving are a part of our perceptual structure.

We consider gravity orientation as a background to perception and to movement. Gravity orientation is integrated into all of the elements of movement. We depend on our own particular orientation to weight and space in order to lift, lean, reach, or meet the other. We use it unconsciously, habitually. To play with this sense of our orientation, to become aware of possible shifts in orientation, can help us move differently and may even help us find new solutions to relational problems.

Gravity orientation helps us find a lowest common denominator for working with any of the structures underlying movement. As we continue with the evolutionary sequence, you will see gravity orientation showing up as a fundamental element of the work.

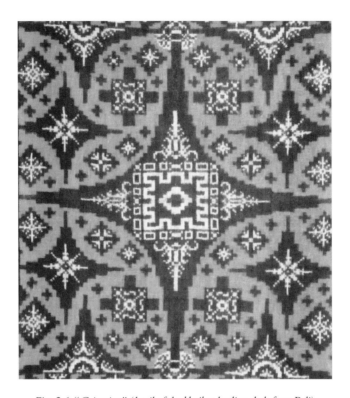

Fig. 2.6. *"Gringsing" (detail of double ikat healing cloth from Bali).*

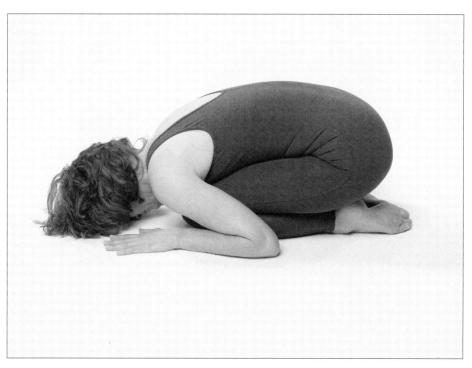

Photograph by John Hession.

CHAPTER 3

Establishing Oneself— the Cell

Movement is organized relative to two directions. One direction is a sense of weight (orientation to ground); the other direction is orientation to space. Each direction supports a person's response to its opposite. After we are born, before we orient to mother or to the breast, we must already have made orientation to gravity. In this early challenge to move, one direction is the weight of one's head, and the other is the sense of mother.

Movement begins as a "pre-movement" in which we make relationship with the Earth's gravity field and to its opposite—our sense of a spatial world. There are different ways for each of us to do this pre-movement, but from the day we leave the womb, we move before we move by relating to gravity and space.

In learning a movement, pre-movement sets the stage for what happens next. People have differences in how they do pre-movement. One person may begin throwing a ball by first establishing his or her stance on the ground, settling back on the heels. Another person may begin the throw by lifting up on the toes, extending the spine, and orienting to the catcher.

The process of learning movement, of changing quality of movement, is really about how we become aware of pre-movement. To find a new pre-movement, we notice new bits of information inside ourselves or in the world around us; we gain a new perception.

We begin with the perception of establishing self. By self, we mean the present time sensations of our body, not the image of our existence or our story. Finding an established sense of self begins by sensing Earth's gravity field, allowing gravity to find us.

ESTABLISHING ONESELF

For a child to reach into the world, he must first feel ready. Being ready to reach out depends upon being established enough in one's sense of body and self. What are the elements of perception and feeling that make up our established sense of self?

How do you establish yourself? Find out what you do to collect yourself, to find ground, to coalesce.

To meet a new challenge, to recover from a startling event, to calm yourself in foreign territory, what do you do?

What have you already done in your mind? Where did you go for a sense of your home, inside?

Discover what establishing yourself means to you. As you imagine establishing yourself, see if

TIMELINE OF LIFE ON EARTH

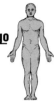

100 Thousand Years Ago
100–150 THOUSAND
Homosapiens

One Million Years Ago
1.5–3 MILLION
Pre-humans, First members of Genus Homo,
African Australopithecines

10 Million Years Ago

 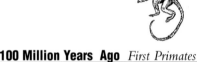 **100 Million Years Ago** *First Primates*
220 MILLION *Mammals*
350 MILLION *Reptiles, First life to rise off the ground.*
360 MILLION *Amphibians, First life in gravity (on land).*
400–500 MILLION *Lancelets and Fish*
550 MILLION *Flatworm/3 tissue layers w. Mesoderm or*
Muscle/connective tissue emergence.
First bilaterally symmetrical life.
630 MILLION *Cnidarians (Coelenterata)/2 tissue layers:*
gut (endoderm) & Neural Net (Ectoderm).
First radially symmetrical life.

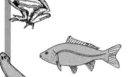

One Billion Years Ago
1.2 BILLION–700 MILLION *Multicellular Animals*
2–1.2 BILLION *Cells in Aggregate, Symbiotic Colonies*
or Endosymbiotic Relationships
2 BILLION *Eukryotic cells (cells with nucleus)*
3.8–3.5 BILLION *First Life on Planet/Prokaryotic cells, bacteria,*
green algae, organelles, rhibosomes. First sphere shaped life.
4.7 BILLION *Birth of Earth*

10 Billion Years Ago
11–20 BILLION *Age of the Universe*
(Big Bang), Birth of space.

Fig. 3.2. *Timeline of Life on Earth.*
(Drawing by Susan Kress Hamilton.)

you can find a movement that fits. Then notice what you sense in your body.

What did you do? What was your strategy? How did your body shape itself? What meaning did you make out of the words, "establish yourself"? Take a moment to notice what you did; write it down, or tell a friend. Then consider the experiences of three movement students:

One student curled up and rocked gently. She reports that to establish herself she needs to be alone and get quiet. Privacy and quiet are important in reestablishing the sense of herself.

Another stood and rubbed his body all over, like one would in a shower. He reports that he finds bodywork helpful when he is stressed. The sense of being touched gives him a feeling of self.

Still another stood up and started to dance, making deep sounds. He reports that he feels happy and good in his body at parties and dances, or taking group hikes into the mountains.

Hearing another person's report of movement impulse gives us a chance to notice other aspects of ourselves, and fine-tune the sense of what we need. Clearly, there are many ways to make meaning out of the invitation to establish yourself. There are many ways to put that meaning into movement.

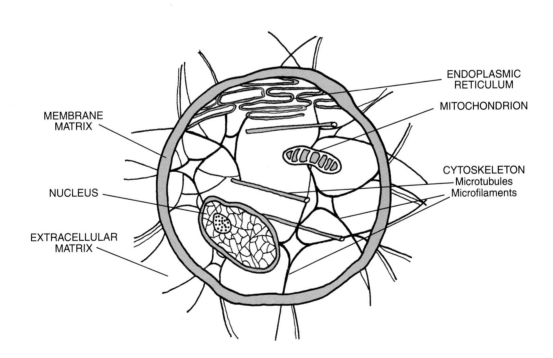

Fig. 3.3. *Basic eukaryote cell.* (Drawing by Susan Kress Hamilton.)

THE EVOLUTIONARY STORY BEGINS WITH THE CELL

We start with the beginning of life on our planet Earth, just as cells have emerged from the primordial ooze. Use the following metaphor of a cell to play with the shape of your body and use imagination, breath, sound, and creative impulse to find your relationship to the story of evolution and to the story of your movement.

We begin the evolutionary story with the cell. With the cell, life takes a definite form. Form, in turn, defines the way movement takes place. We look at the cell, and other forms of life, to help us to explore our perception of our body. How does our form define the way we move? What happens if we play with our sense of form, simplify it?

The first cells came into existence between 3.5 and 3.8 billion years ago. For at least 1.5 billion years life only took the form of single cells. It was a durable, simple, and persistent form. Multi-celled organisms can reliably be said to have existed for only the last billion years. We are multi-celled organisms. And we are made of single cells.

The particular cell we are going to consider is the *eukaryote* cell. These are more complex than their predecessors. They have a true nucleus. Eukaryotes are the form of cells that make up all the plants and animals of our world.

The cell is, most importantly, a way of describing how biology distinguishes self and other. Within the cell are organelles that enable a cell to have an existence distinct from other cells. In particular we want to focus on two elements of the eukaryotic cell. These two elements make the cell separate and give it a sense of weight and space. First, there is a nucleus, containing genetic material. The cell's identity is defined, in part, by this genetic code that helps determine its individual personality. Each of us has our individuality in movement. Then there is something called a cytoskeleton. This gives the cell a very basic gravity orientation. Contained within this cytoskeleton is a microtubule matrix. This microtubule matrix has been called the nervous system of the cell.[1,2]

The microtubules within the cytoskeleton are gravity sensitive.[3] They orient to gravity, to Earth. Every cell in our body knows gravity through its microtubules. We can also say that cells are opportunistic to space, that cells adapt to space. Cells use and occupy extracellular space, and in so doing change their shape accordingly. Cells orient to space.[4] We also orient to space, and change our shape accordingly.

The form of a cell is both simple and complex. We have alluded to the complexity. The simplicity is found in the basic concept of the cell. It is formed in the impulse to define separateness. The contents of each cell are surrounded and contained by a selectively semi-permeable membrane. This membrane separates cell from matrix. The word matrix derives from the Latin word for mother. The cell's matrix is an intercellular soup. In becoming separate, the cell has done so securely surrounded by its mother.

The cell has a defined boundary. Outside is other. Inside is self. This true statement is also false—the cell never loses its interpenetration with its environment. Parts of the cytoskeleton within the cell also extend through the cell membrane and out as a web in the matrix around the cell. A cell is both separate from and a part of its web.

As a movement exercise, imagine what it feels like to be a single cell. Use images of cells, along with other perceptual cues, to enter into your body's version of pretending to be a single cell. It is possible to empathize with the metaphor of the single cell; it is a story that takes place within your body.

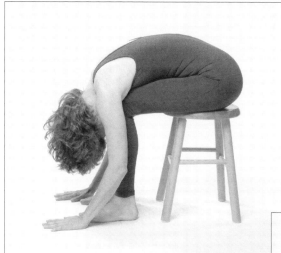

Fig. 3.4. *Seated cell exploration.*
(Photograph by John Hession.)

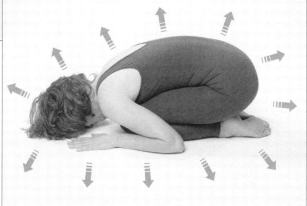

Fig. 3.5. *Breathing omni-directionally.*
(Photograph by John Hession.)

Find a roughly spherical posture: either the deep fold (the child's pose in yoga), or sitting in a chair with the head and shoulders hanging over your legs, your belly resting on your lap. (Use pillows on your lap if it helps you to relax your torso.)

Let your abdomen relax. Rest into gravity. Notice your breath for a while. Imagine breathing through the skin of your whole body. Cells breathe in all directions. Breathe into the volume of the body, so you feel expansion of the front and back and sides of the body. Explore the sense of breathing spherically.

The cell is filled with fluid (as is the human body). Imagine you can feel the weight and motion of the fluid within you.

Notice the sense of weight, of internal context, whether the abdomen can be soft. What is it like to feel boundary—the skin—and within it a fluid matrix?

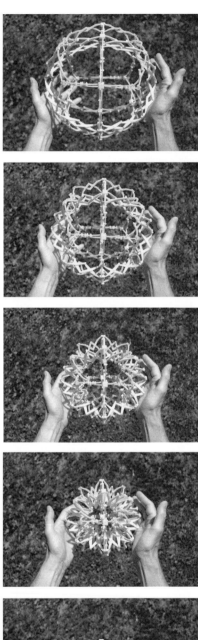

Figs.3.6a,b,c,d,e. *Playing with expansion toy to see and feel omni-directional orientation and breath.*

If a partner is available, have him or her use the hands to provide touch in the low back, upper buttocks, mid-back, upper back. If no partner is handy, use your own hands as far as you can reach. The hand pressure can let you know where you are trying to breathe and confirm that the breath is moving into the back.

Breath is part of the cell experience. This is a chance to breathe with a sense that the breath moves backward toward the spine and downward into the bottom of the pelvis. After you find these dimensions of breath, see if you can feel that the breath moves in all directions within the body. The cell is spherical. There are no corners or front and back. The cell breath is omni-directional. Are there any directions that could be amplified to find this omni-directional sense of breath through the entire surface of your skin? Can you "touch" and establish the volume of yourself with cell breath?

Can you "hear" your breath in all directions? Is listening to your breath helpful in establishing either more weight or spaciousness?

After you try this exercise, reflect on your response to it. There isn't any correct response. Does it immediately grab your imagination, leading you into an engaging experience? Or does it seem trivial, or hard to enter into? How did you make sense out of the instructions? Is your experience new or does it remind you of some previous experience?

TRANSITION

We have met and embodied the cell. We will add complexity to form and to movement and experience the movement of each step as we do so. At the same time, we refer always to our ability to establish ourselves, have a boundary, a sense of weight, and to find the complementary perception—a sense of spatial orientation. This balance of awareness, inside and outside, up and down, is a constant for life on our planet and for our movement curriculum.

NOTES FOR TEACHERS AND BODY THERAPISTS ON USING THE CONCEPT OF CELL

You can use the concept of Cell to help clients locate their body and feel contained. People dealing with nervousness or fright may find this calming. Cell is a sanctuary for a felt sense of whole body, for the profundity of simply being. In a class setting, Cell can provide a baseline at the beginning, middle, or end of a class, and can provide continuity in a series of classes.

Cell is also useful for people suffering from back pain. Hip flexors can slacken; back muscles are gently stretched; the abdomen can be soft; attention is given to the sensations and movements in the surface of the back.

The Cell experience, on the bodywork table, on a chair, or draped over a physioball, is a useful resource for relieving back pain. It provides an opportunity to help someone soothe and settle.

The key to using Cell or any of the suggested movement exercises is the practitioner's familiarity with this kind of experience in his or her own body. Empathy, the capacity to track the changes in a client, is informed by the capacity to track perceptions inside oneself.

The value of Cell stems in part from bringing the hip flexors, the psoas, and iliacus into a position of least challenge. When the body is folded up, hip flexors, erector spinae, belly wall, and head can all begin to sense rest.

Rest, our birthright, eludes human beings. Most of us need to relearn how to truly rest. The level of flight-or-fight reaction that lives in our body requires considerable attention to undo. Levine has spoken of the "tuned" autonomic nervous system, meaning an autonomic nervous system that has lost the ability to return to a normal, neutral state.[5] Somatic therapy, holistic bodywork, and perceptual approaches to movement are ways to relieve some of the stress that comes from chronic sympathetic arousal.

Each time a client explores Cell, there is an opportunity to sense feedback from the body. One may notice the degree of relaxation that happens in the muscles, the speed with which a felt sense of weight arrives, the amount of depth and volume that is noticeable when one breathes. In this way, one grows a capacity to establish groundedness, and a felt sense of boundary.

People with acute levels of arousal, with a history of trauma, may need guidance and support from a competent practitioner. However, the exercise is simple and can be done at home. The ability to find support for oneself in this posture contradicts a learned sense of helplessness and collapse. A true posture of containment and softening ironically builds a self that can move out of collapse.

From an osteopathic point of view, Cell allows spasming hip flexor muscles to release in a manner consistent with Jones's theory of counterstrain.[6] As hip flexors and belly wall release, the body is in a position for the back, buttock, and neck muscles to relax as well, especially as the student learns to find an easy quality of breath into the low back and sacral areas.

Another osteopathic concept is motility—the intrinsic fluid movement within the body. Cell is an opportunity to notice the sense that the largely fluid contents of the body are in motion, are continuously moving independently of our gross motor activity. As we breathe omni-directionally, we may also listen to the motion that is present. Noticing the motion that is present can be deeply soothing and healing.

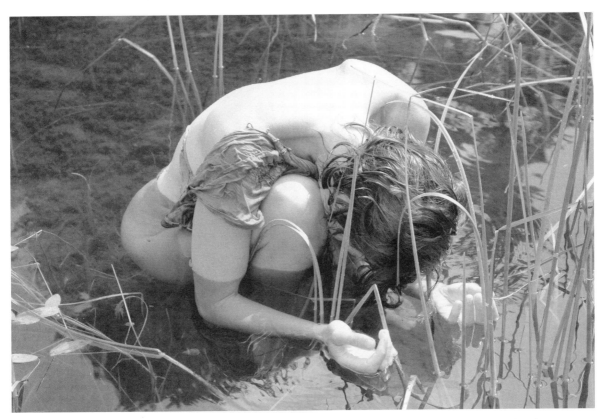

Photograph by John Hession.

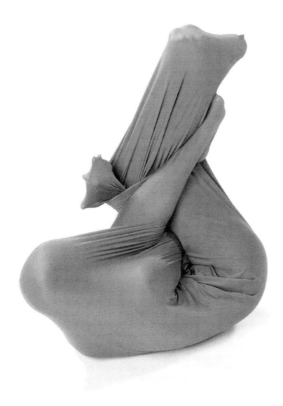

Fig. 4.1. Photograph by John Hession.

CHAPTER 4

The Cell's Contents and Container—
Cell Movement and Boundary

In this chapter, we explore the sensation of our surface, our fluid volume, and a moment-to-moment surrendering to weight. We begin by focusing on boundaries. We then use the metaphor of the moving cell to help us learn about shifting perception from inside to outside, and defining the place where these two come together. This work begins our orientation to the world outside.

NOTICING YOUR BOUNDARY

What arises when you hear the word *boundary*? Do you imagine the state line on a cross-country trip, or the fence that separates your property from your neighbor's? Do you think about your interpersonal boundaries, where your space stops and another person's space begins? What about your ability to say no or ask for what you need? This line of inquiry helps us establish ourselves. To establish ourselves in the world, we need to feel the place where our edge meets other.

Write down, draw, or move a story in your life about boundaries. After you find some boundary story, ask yourself how your body felt or acted in the story, or how someone else's body behaved in the story. Think about what you do in your imagination, or in action, or in body awareness

that lets you feel a sense of boundary. Then move, sense, or imagine the boundary quality that you found.

Here are some boundary stories of other students:

A medical student describes her experience working in an inner-city emergency room. *"The boundary issue was really up for me as soon as I was doing rotations. This is a picture of me (describes drawing) in the ER with the docs, the PAs, the nurses, and the patients. I'm the tall oval shape with the black jagged line around it. Outside the black line you can see a light pink. That's the kind part of me that I let out for patients and some of the nurses who have been nice to me. The black jagged lines are strong to keep out the humiliation and so people can't see if I'm nervous. Inside the oval is a tangle of red lines. But that isn't about my boundary. I put on that black jagged line when I go to the hospital. It takes me a while to let it down when I get home. I stroke my cat and he licks my hand. This is a picture of me, and my cat. There is a thick blue layer of color around both of us and around the apartment."*

As the med student looks at her drawing she senses her elbows wanting to jab people who get too close to her. She moves her elbow sharply out to the side and she purses her lips slightly at the same time.

A young man reports that ex-girlfriends tell him he doesn't have "good boundaries." He knows that he is friendly around women. *"I don't know what a good boundary is supposed to be,"* he says. *"Does it mean I should be more cautious, and less eager to reach out? I was quite cautious with a woman and she complained the most about what happened. If you ask me to draw or move or show my boundary, it feels like I am trying to contain what my impulses are."* The notion of boundaries is a puzzle for this fellow. He reports a vague dizziness when asked about how the sense of boundary shows up in his body.

One woman talks about how she has a well-developed sense of "mine versus yours." This woman lived communally for a long time. *"If I was making some lunch and someone came in the house who wasn't my guest, I didn't offer them anything to eat. If someone else put some food in the fridge, I didn't touch it. I wouldn't smile at a man unless I wanted to get to know him at an intimate level. I posted a note when I wanted to take a shower and I was out of there, with the tub wiped down, on the dot of when I was supposed to be. Communal living goes great with people who aren't sloppy about living within their lines."* She reports a feeling of satisfaction in her legs and belly, and warmth, when she reflected on her strategy.

CELL BOUNDARY

Boundaries are complex. We experiment with boundary issues in many of the exercises. Whether for good or ill, life concerns itself with defining inside and outside. Is it possible to reexamine our human adaptations to this dilemma?

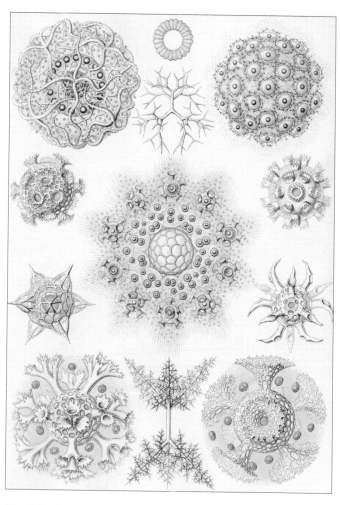

Fig. 4.2. *Varieties of cell shapes as drawn by Ernst Haekel.* (From Haeckel's *Art Forms in Nature.*)

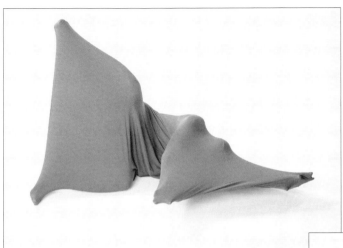

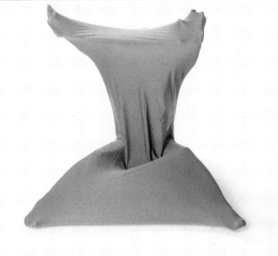

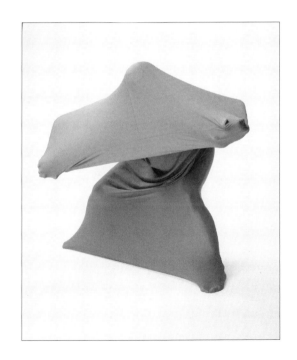

Figs. 4.3a,b,c. *Exploring boundary and flow.*
(Photographs by John Hession.)

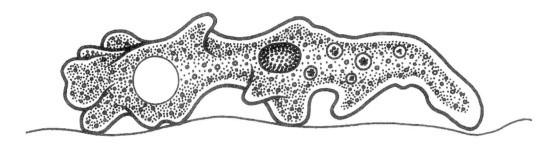

The cell gives us a context to move and sense the boundary of our body in a relatively simple way.

Cells have many shapes. We started with the spherical shape because it has an important quality for movement. A sphere is an omni-directional potential of action. It has an omni-directional orientation. A sphere can be thought of as a place of all possibilities, a place of creative abundance. But cells can come in a very broad spectrum of shapes. The unusual drawings by Haeckel illustrate some of the shapes that single cells come in.

Some cells can change their shape. In order to move, cells can extend parts of their membrane to create pseudopods. The pseudopods fill with cytoplasm and cytoskeleton. At the same time the pseudopods assist the cell in movement. In order

to change shape, the cell must be plastic in its membrane, and fluidic in its contents.

The cell has a selectively semi-permeable membrane. Imagine a wrapper that is alive and intelligent. It is a gatekeeper in both directions, like a customs station at a country's border. It decides moment to moment, like the immune system decides, what constitutes self and other. What belongs inside me, what belongs outside?

The contents of a cell are both structural and fluid. The cell has a stable shape, and it is mutable within certain limits.

Fig. 4.4 above. *Amoeba with pseudopods that form and dissolve as it flows along.* (Reproduced with permission from Buchsbaum, R., Buchsbaum, M., Pearse, V., and Pearse, J., *Animals Without Backbones: An Introduction to the Invertebrates,* Third Edition. Chicago: University of Chicago Press, 1987, p. 25.)

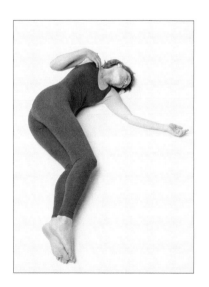
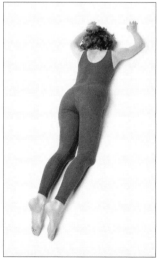
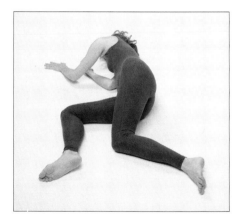

Lie supine with your knees flexed and your feet on the floor. Imagine the fluid fullness of the cell body as your liquid ballast. Initiate a roll on to one side, imagining that the ballast is pouring very slowly into its lowest point. Play with pouring the contents of the cell body in the head, the trunk, and the pelvis, allowing the limbs to drop and spill as necessary while the axial part of the body pours.

Roll the weighted, fluid-filled container of your body, and notice the outside of each part of your container as it contacts the floor. Examine the sensations of contact slowly rolling. Use different positions to assist the rolling of the skull part of the container. Take the time to explore, in sensation, the curvature of the skull—the top and sides and back of the skull, and the transitions between each of these parts.

A helpful image is that of a hard-boiled egg. Your skin and soft tissue is the egg's shell. Imagine that as you roll the egg on a hard surface, the egg is slowly cracked until the entire shell is riddled with fissures. In this way the shell reveals its flexible soft insides. The sense of body transforms from hard separate parts to a sense that the entire body is equanimous—in full control—and whole.

Return to rolling the contents and observe how slow pouring has changed, especially in the head. Does the head have the same quality of weight as the other body segments (trunk and pelvis)? Allow your mouth to open slightly and relax your pelvic floor. This will give more sense of dropped weight for the head.

Figs. 4.5a,b,c,d,e,f below. *Rolling and pouring, sensing the skin, allowing weight to meet ground.* (Photographs by John Hession.)

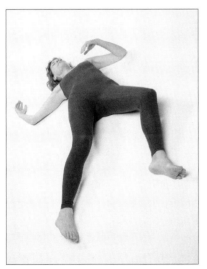
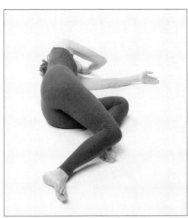
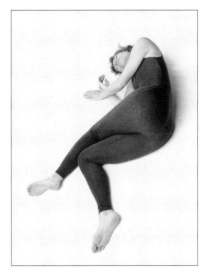

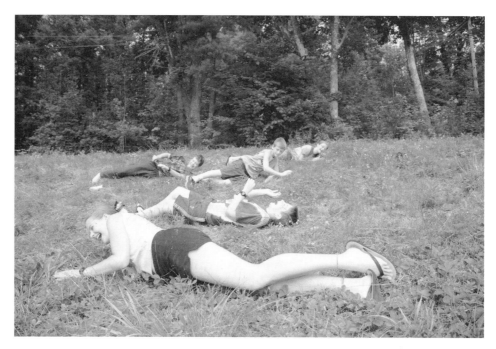

Fig. 4.6. *Children rolling down a hill.*

Experiment so that you find a speed of rolling that is comfortable. If you get to a "stuck" point, pause, reestablish an omni-directional breath, and notice what happens. Some may find a very slow roll is most informative. Others may need to roll quickly in the way we all rolled down a hill when we were young.

NOTES FOR TEACHERS
AND BODY THERAPISTS ON
ROLLING AND POURING

The Pouring exercise allows the body to move and feel contact with an external context through the sense of boundary (skin, scalp, and clothing). Most people don't have a learned capacity to notice feeling the surfaces of their body. Noticing skin or scalp immediately amplifies a sense of body, and gives the brain information on the shape and position of the body in space.

If people don't want to get on the floor, have them pour themselves into their seat and legs as they sit up from either the cell shape on the chair or getting out of bed in the morning. It's also possible to establish a sense of omni-directionality of the skull surface by rolling and pouring the head on the wall.

The sense of rolling and pouring allows people to track the sense of weight as they move. This enables them to notice where the sense of weight may be missing, and adjust movement so that the sense of weight improves.

We began rolling and pouring with boundaries. Psychological boundaries are linked to sensory and perceptual boundaries. Rolling and pouring teaches us, through sense perception, that we have a tangible membrane that surrounds us. This experience can be a resource in situations in which we must establish a sense of self—situations that are inhibiting, that cause us to lose the sense of who we are or what we feel. We can also become overfocused on our internal experience to the exclusion of noticing the space around us. Godard suggests that working with the sense of skin shifts the quality of a person's movement even when his or her true proprioceptive sense is impaired.[1] If we pinch the student's skin, for instance on the middle of his or her back, and ask the student to move by drawing the skin out of our hand, the movement becomes more economical and graceful. We call this proprioceptive-like because technically sensations in the skin are not considered part of the proprioceptive system.

In somatic therapy, it is useful to help clients learn to feel their skin. A client recalling trauma, or in some other way sympathetically aroused, can use the sense of skin as a psychological anchor. Feeling the sense of one's physical boundary brings one into present time. It establishes one's location in space directly and efficiently.

Emotional disturbance from past trauma draws its power from a remembered event. The client is living in a temporal (time-based) state of disorientation. The tendency to be overwhelmed by temporal disorientation is balanced by establishing the body in space. We can establish ourselves in space through the experience of our skin, feeling as much of the surface of our skin as possible, and feeling our movement guided by the sense of skin.

Using a sense of skin to shift the quality of movement and the autonomic state in clients and students can be experientially verified. Rolling and pouring is a way of finding the sense of boundary and amplifying our skill for recalling it.

The skin boundary, the cell membrane, is the edge from which we consider the world outside us. We have established ourselves, and have heightened the boundary between self and other, by feeling gravity and the ground in our movement. The next step is to extend our sense of the outer world beyond our skin.

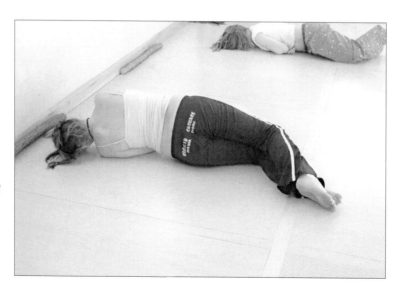

Fig. 4.7. *Students rolling and pouring in movement class.*

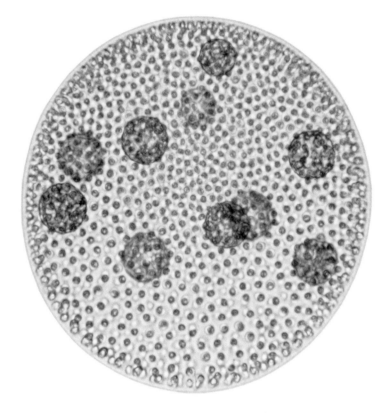

Fig. 5.1. *Volvox green algae colony.*
(Reproduced with permission from Dr. James W. Richardson/Visuals Unlimited.)

CHAPTER 5

The Cell Moves in Its Matrix — Cell Colony

A cell contains a fluid matrix. A fluid matrix also surrounds it. By *fluid matrix* we mean the ocean of water-based liquid that all cells live in. Cells don't live in isolation. This simple fact offers a lesson about our lives: Living creatures are tender and vulnerable and only thrive in situations that offer supportive context. If a person stops feeling connected to community and world, he or she will not thrive. Humans can feel disconnected even when they are not, in fact, alone. There is a difference between having a matrix and experiencing that one has a matrix. The latter is more important because we are so affected by what we perceive.

Context shapes our movements. The space we move in is pregnant with the meaning we make. Our pre-movement involves how we sense our self and is determined by qualities that we sense consciously or unconsciously in our environment. The third step in the evolutionary story is the bridge between sense of self and sense of context. What do we mean by context and how can we use the sense of context to shift the quality of our movement?

FINDING CONNECTION TO MATRIX

How do you find a sense of matrix? Start by grounding the abstraction, "matrix." We describe the intercellular and intracellular matrix as being a living network that connects all parts of the cell to the soup in which the cell floats. This intracellular web also connects to neighboring cells. If you applied this relationship to the way people live, how would this metaphor translate?

Human beings have telephones, postal services, and Internet connections. We have neighborhoods. We have families, friends, pets, business associates, or colleagues with whom we act out the stories of our lives.

People also feel relationship to the Earth, the sky, God or spirit, or nature. Each time we breathe, we take plant breath into us and give back our breath. When we eat, we take creatures and plants into our body and then give most of it back.

People pray or meditate or practice ritual. We have clubs, associations, sporting events, even television.

Does any or all of this constitute matrix?

Matrix can mean mother, or the substance that holds us and nurtures us, as mothers do. The cell derives oxygen from its matrix. It depends on the matrix for information, for support in all its forms and activities. For a human, the felt sense of connectedness can be matrix. The sense of support, of being in communion, can be the most important support and motivation in our lives.

Emilie Conrad, the creator of Continuum™, mentions that Oscar Ichazo said all search for consciousness is about mother loss. Emilie believes it's more appropriate to say "matrix loss.[1]" In other words, we all search for a context big enough, intelligent enough, and loving enough that we will feel reassured and at peace.

Consider what your sense of matrix is.

What is your relationship to matrix? How do you find it? How do you avoid finding it, if that's what you do? Think of an example in your life where you are acting, or moving, or noticing relationship to matrix.

What did you find out? Compare your discovery with the experience of these three people:

One woman associates matrix with gatherings in her family's country home. The large group of relatives elicits for her a sense of belonging, a sense of being part of something bigger that is friendly and inclusive. At the end of a warm summer afternoon, she lies in the grass with her niece and watches the clouds, secure in the knowledge that everyone she loves is nearby.

Another person feels best when he's doing a hundred-mile ride with some of his bicycle buddies. He loves being in a pack of men pumping their legs until they can almost pump no more, of feeling the challenging workout while the scenery rolls by; thoughts diminish, anxieties diminish. That is how he senses belonging, a sense of immediacy.

A woman remembers giving birth as a time when there was no doubt about who she was and why she was alive. She felt the

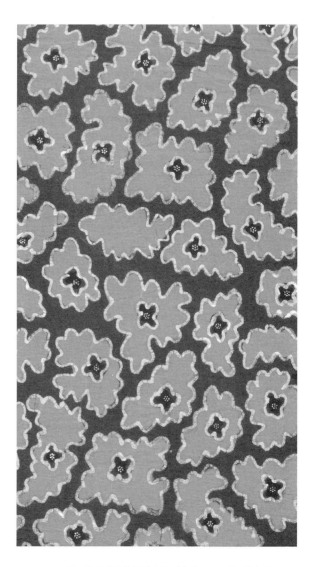

Fig. 5.2. *"Cells" (detail of Indonesian textile).*

invisible presence of other beings that were with her, supporting her. During pregnancy, she never felt alone. There was a being inside her that knew her at a silent level and that she recognized as seeing her, as being in harmony with her. Her daughter has gone on to find other sources of belonging and this mother loves the moments that they can still cuddle and lose the sense of separateness.

What do these stories do to your sense of matrix?

Now think about how you feel in proximity to other people. Can you both feel your sense of self and feel a sense of others being near you? Does the same felt sense of matrix that arises in an ideal circumstance speak to you when you are in a group of people? Notice what comes up; note it for later.

THE CELL COLONY

There are many evolutionary pathways that led from the single eukaryote cells (collectively known as protozoa) to multi-celled organisms (collectively known as metazoa).[2] The fossil records are ambiguous about the next step from single cell. In present time, however, there is a creature that illustrates one way that single cells have come together to form something new. It is a cell colony called Volvox, composed of flagellate green algae cells (protozoa) that stay together after dividing from the mother cell.

What is the movement from individuality to cooperative association? Each of us faces this movement in our development. Over a billion years ago, this possibility emerged. Starting with colonies of identical daughter cells, cells eventually gained the capacity to differentiate into separate tissues with different functions. This was an important step from single, free-living cells to complex multicellular animals.

In the cell colony, individual cells are mysteriously linked together so the group of cells functions as a single entity. It's hard to imagine human beings performing such a complex and cooperative ballet. Wagon trains crossing the frontier together, basketball teams moving down a court—neither of these examples express the simplicity of cooperation and association of the cell colony. Herds of migrating grazing animals, colonies of ants and termites, flocks of geese taking flight, schools of fish moving synchronously—these examples are closer to illustrating the quality of coordinated movement that the cell colony pioneered.

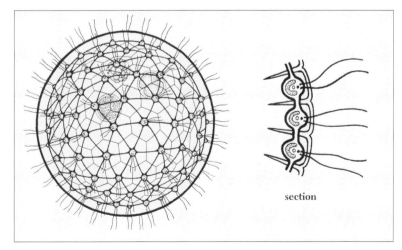

Fig. 5.3. *Diagram of Volvox protozoan cell colony. The outer cells have two flagella, and this colony can actively swim.* (Reproduced with permission from Buchsbaum, R., Buchsbaum, M., Pearse, V., and Pearse, J., *Animals Without Backbones: An Introduction to the Invertebrates*, Third Edition. Chicago: University of Chicago Press, 1987, p. 43.)

section

How does this coordination take place? What allows a colony of cells with identical DNA to do what most human committees cannot—that is, efficiently and mysteriously work together to move in a common direction, each member providing precisely the right contribution of flagella response so that the whole colony moves together?

The Volvox story is a pivotal place in the evolutionary story in which we observe entrainment. There is resonance and communication among the cells. This phenomenon presently exceeds the ability of science to explain it. In fact, there is very little that explains herd and flock behavior because these behaviors also seem to depend on a resonance difficult to measure.

This resonance, the ability to relate harmoniously, can be demonstrated between the soundboards of musical instruments, or between magnetic devices. Until recently it was not a phenomenon that science accepted as occurring between living creatures. Still, the Volvox story is a simple example of resonant behavior.

A Group Exercise: ENTRAINMENT THROUGH RESONANCE

The phenomenon of entrainment can be explored in a movement class.

Divide into two groups (of four or more). The groups take turns moving and observing. Members of the moving group close their eyes and begin to move near each other but not touching. They are directed to follow their impulses to move fast or slow, big or small, and in any fashion that suits their mood or inspiration. The second group just observes for five to ten minutes. The groups then exchange roles. To add to the fun, replay the exercise and tell people to move in as individual a way as possible.

We predict that in both instances, even if you invite intentional individuality, after a few minutes you will see uncanny patterns of similarity. We don't attempt to explain why this happens. Rather we invite you to keep the question open as we visit the evolutionary mystery once again.

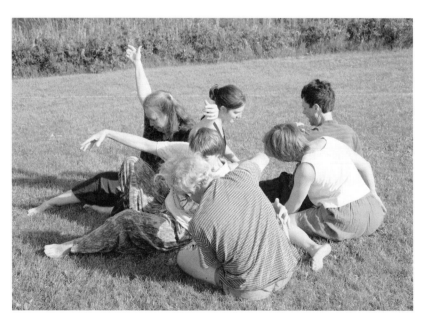

Figs. 5.4 and 5.5.
At right and opposite page:
Cell colony exercise: moving in proximity, with inclusive attention.
(Photographs by John Hession.)

Looking at the simple protozoan cell colony gives us an example of resonant behavior that leaves out such complexities as a nervous system, differentiated tissue, or any of the other factors we would have to consider in a higher animal or a human. We are left with the naked mystery of how simple cells are able to coordinate with each other when there are no visible means of communication and no visible source of collective intelligence.

Cell Colony is a group activity. A group of six or more is preferable.

Begin by establishing a sense of being one single cell. In the deep fold, find the sense of volume using breath. Find the sense of the cell membrane by pouring and rolling slowly on the floor. Using the motion of rolling and pouring, establish your separate space from other members of the group.

Notice your own cell body, and begin to inclusively attend to the space around you, omni-directionally. *Inclusive attention*[3] means noticing one's established sense of self and, at the same time, noticing that which is outside oneself— other people, the surrounding space, the objects in one's environment. It is harder to pay attention to something in front of us and at the same time feel equally aware of what is to the side of us or behind us. Establishing a sense of cell body helps enable us to find an omni-directional quality of awareness in different situations. Another way to say this is that we are establishing a sense of omni-directional orientation.

Notice your preference for feeling your body or noticing others nearby. Your preference to feel yourself or to pay attention to others near you is a clue to how you initiate movement. In different

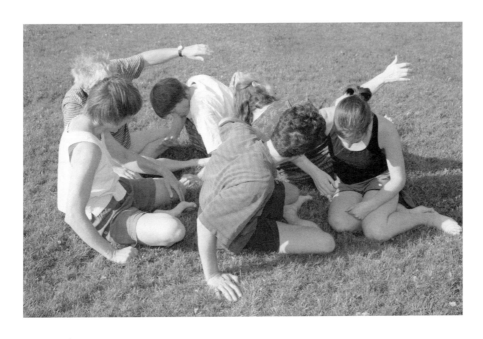

movement exercises you may notice that your awareness of what you feel changes. Each context, the meaning and circumstances of a movement, affects how our pre-movement is set up.

Start to roll and pour your cell body. How does your sense of proximity to others shift? Feel the potency of the space between you and others. Try to feel how the potency shifts with the changes in distance. How does noticing the space and the other participants change how you can feel the surface of your own body, your weight, your volume, and your breath?

Now, as a group, slowly roll closer to one another. Continue to roll nearer until the distance separating you is small but you are not physically touching. Again, feel what this does to the sense of inclusive attention. Do you feel yourself or what is outside you more strongly? Are you comfortable with this level of proximity? Proximity is a form of touch. As a reenactment of the colonial protozoa, you are in a position to notice what proximity to others means to your body. The meaning may be felt as pleasure, anxiety, curiosity, or any number of other experiences.

Act on what you notice. If you feel curious, continue to move in slight rolling or other fluid-like ways, feeling the potency of close proximity, what your body can sense at a primitive level. If you feel uncomfortable with being near to others, slowly roll away, noticing how your comfort level changes with each stage of rolling away.

For those who have stayed in close proximity, you are invited to move, as a group, in a designated direction. Move by rolling, or wiggling, noting that flagellate protozoa (like those in a Volvox cell colony) have flagella and are able to propel the raft of their collective bodies with these waving tails. Find out what it takes to be inclusively attentive to one's own sense of cell as well as an omni-directional awareness of the group and the space into which the group moves.

Those who have moved away from the clump of cell bodies are invited to inclusively attend as well, either by maintaining a comfortable distance to the group through movement, or by noticing how the movement of the group toward or away from oneself changes the felt sense.

Wherever you happen to be, open yourself to any and all sensations, feelings, images, or meaning-making that may occur to you. Let your attention be open and unmanaged. What do you notice?

Remember your earlier experience with matrix, and your sense of feeling your self in proximity to others. What is your body telling you about matrix now?

Now pour yourself onto your hands and feet and pour yourself into your feet and legs to stand up. Start to walk in and out of the empty spaces of the group, as a walking human. Notice your sense of fluid-filled body as you walk. Enjoy the flow of your walk, noticing the possibility of omni-directional orientation. Then play with a sense of colonizing the space by noticing the other people walking. Is it possible to notice your own volume and container while simultaneously noticing others?

Consider the proposition that resonance, at the cellular level or in people, is a natural consequence of omni-directional orientation, an attention field that is inclusive to inside and outside in all directions.

THE CELL COLONY IN EVOLUTION

Cells teamed up to be a cell colony. They worked together as the precursor to a multi-celled organism. In the next chapter we explore one of the ways that cells made the transition to being a multi-celled creature with differentiated tissue.

NOTES FOR TEACHERS AND BODY THERAPISTS ON CELL COLONY

The Cell Colony exercise is a complex and extended use of metaphor. It focuses on a stage of evolution that is not well known. Fossils from the Pre-Cambrian era don't tell the story of the first protozoan colonies with any clarity. Most scientists agree that an organism like Volvox was a likely part of the process from single- to multi-cellular life. How do living creatures coordinate their movement with each other? How did flagellate protozoa learn to move together and begin to differentiate roles?

As students of movement, Cell Colony is the step in which we experience inclusive attention, the capacity to feel two directions of attention at the same time. The students sensitize themselves to perceptions of space—the sense of potent space. When the space holds another, students ask themselves how the other changes their ability to stay established in their own experience.

Cell Colony can be used repeatedly with an ongoing movement study group. Inclusive attention is a skill that can be practiced and this exercise provides a playful and stimulating context for doing so. Opening to an experience of matrix is not a skill, but in practicing inclusive attention sensing matrix can occur as a happy accident.

Cell Colony brings the student closer to the origins of cellular cooperation and communication. Without coordination and cooperation among cells, multi-celled organisms could not exist. Similarly, all higher forms of life must live within a larger context of species and the ecosystem that supports that species.

We need to sense our resonance with our community and all the less visible aspects of everything implied by matrix. Sensing matrix lets in the impression of proximity, and allows us to feel the field of awareness that surrounds our body. In the absence of this, our ability to reach out physically is inhibited. The perception of our surroundings is necessary for fully coordinated movement.

Optimal coordination of movement requires the perception of what is around, above, and outside of us. If coordination is impaired by this missing perception, it is helpful to be able to recognize this, and offer a remedy. We can grow in the capacity to feel the space around us. It helps to become aware that the meanings we make of space, or the people or things around us, shape our perception of space. If we recognize the meanings we hold and become skilled in the use of sensation, imagination, and movement, we can change the way we perceive; we can make important changes in the qualities of our movement. Cell Colony supports this exploration.

Some students may notice that to feel comfortable they move their body away from the group. Students may then judge themselves as lacking the capacity for intimacy. It is important to point out that acknowledging the level of proximity that is truly comfortable is the beginning of self-organization and regulation of health. By noticing what is true for us, we can be spatially far but relationally present because a key barrier to relationship has been removed. Often our greatest barrier to health is an image of what should be. We encourage an inquiry into what is true in the absence of judgments and self-image.

In this chapter we help the student to notice omni-directional orientation. This type of orientation is kinespheric. *Kinesphere* describes the shape of the attentional field that surrounds our body. It is a useful concept because so much of physical and psychological therapy, especially trauma work, concentrates on rebuilding the missing aspects of the client's kinesphere. For example, someone who received a blow to the head may not have the ability to feel the space to that side of the head. This profoundly affects the person's movement and ability to function, but may lie hidden until the practitioner starts to look at the client's perceptual structure— in this case, the missing place of kinesphere.

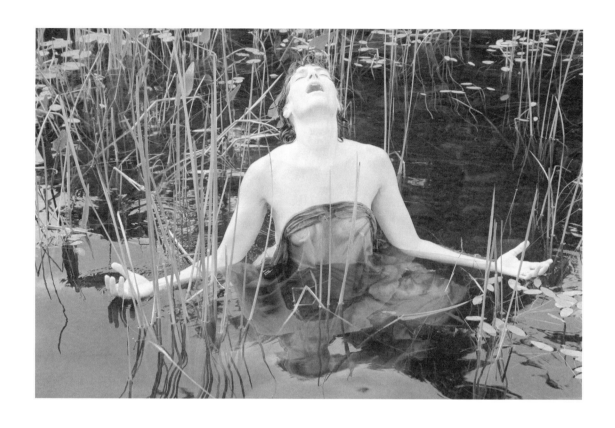

CHAPTER 6

Vessel—the Primitive Gut Body

CELLS AS PART OF A NEW WHOLE

Cell colonies are aggregates of cells working together and acting like one big organism, while still being made up of individual cells. At some point, however, cells became part of a true multi-celled whole. One of these multi-celled organisms began to create a chamber in which outside was brought within. This led to a new animal shape, one in which there emerged a new function—the primordial gut body.

CONSIDERING THE MATTER OF HAVING A GUT

The human body has a gut tube that begins with the lips and mouth and ends with the rectum and anus. The whole tube passes food from outside, through the body, so that we absorb some of it, but maintains a separation between outside and inside the organism.

Many issues arise when we think about the gut. Our culture uses the phrase "gut feeling;" we feel "sick with worry" or "gutsy." Feeding and sucking arise as issues for every newborn. We also learn to use our mouths to indicate pleasure and pain or discomfort. From childhood's earliest

hour the mouth gets a lot of attention. So does the anus. There is the matter of how our belly feels, whether gas is pressing from inside and causing discomfort, or whether our "gut feelings" indicate safety and pleasure, or fear and disgust.

All complex creatures, those beyond the level of cell colonies, have guts. First, consider the human point of view.

What does the gut body mean to you? When you hear the word gut, what association occurs?

Draw your food tube, or gut body. Label your picture with some notes describing how you feel about different parts of the gut body.

Move the parts of your body in your drawing. Be imaginative. Some of what you draw may not feel independently movable, at least not something you can move on purpose. Just give your body a chance to play with a gut movement of some sort. Pause to notice if you have any mental commentary. Add these comments to your drawing.

Imagine a sound that your gut tube might make while you move it. What kind of sound-track would accompany your drawing or the movements you play with? What creature sound would come out of your gut body?

Use vowels and consonants to note the sound on your drawing. You might put a dialogue bubble

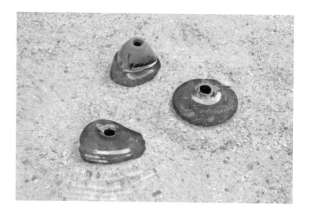

Fig.6.2. *Vessels swallowing water.*

around the sound, as though the gut body is speaking in a comic strip.

Continue to attend openly to your gut. Write some observations about what your gut, or some part of your gut tube, means to you.

After you have noticed your gut story, consider the experiences of other people:

One person reports the following: *"I don't usually spend time thinking about my gut, unless I'm constipated or really hungry. When I drew the gut tube, I realized I have very little idea of what the thing looks like. There is a round shape where my stomach is, and a tube that wraps around like a bunched-up garden hose—that's my intestines. My mouth at the top is wide open and I have labeled it 'too big.' At the bottom is a hole for my anus. I labeled it 'output.' I used yellow, red, and green to show the top of the tube and brown at the end of it. When I tried to move the mouth, I had fun making different expressions with it. I also tried moving my stomach and that was not easy. I pushed my stomach out and tried to roll it around like a belly dancer."*

Another person talks about her experience with the gut body idea: *"First, let me say that this is a very intense question, this gut body business. My mother was a fashion model. She taught her children to hold their bodies in a certain way. It looked like this....(She walks back and forth imitating her mother. Her buttocks are tightened, and her abdomen is held flat, as she walks with a quality of being tall and aloof.) Gut body doesn't enter into the equation! You certainly didn't get the message that eating was something to indulge in.*

"I was living with chronic fatigue-fibromyalgia for several years. I started to understand that my health starts with what I put in my gut, how I feel about it, and how much I let my gut feelings tell me to rest. This has turned the whole gut thing around. I'm still working on letting my belly relax, since my Rolfing lessons and the primitive movement classes. But my back feels better when I do so."

How does your story compare to the two you have just read? Let yourself consider the gut body stories of people you know and see every day. Consider all the issues that revolve around the gut body. Then consider the primitive roots of the human gut body story.

THE VESSEL

The next innovation in the evolutionary story has to do with getting and digesting food. Once cells clustered together in a cooperative blob, an early level of role division became possible. Some cells were at the "front" end of the blob and others were at the "rear." Cells on the outside were using their flagella for propulsion of the group. Somehow the cells moved as a rotating mass, in a particular direction.

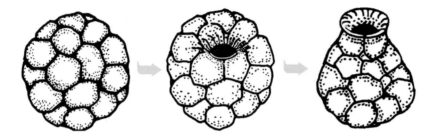

Fig.6.3. *Imagining the steps of shape change. A blob of cells gradually invaginates to become a vessel.* (Drawing by Susan Kress Hamilton.)

THE CELL CLUSTER INVAGINATES

The cell cluster took a big step. A new shape appeared—an invagination was now present. The metaphor of this moment of transformation in shape allows us to re-embody our gut.

Imagine a cluster of cells. Then imagine the cluster is hollowed out, or invaginated. The cluster has now formed a chamber. This leads us to the primordial vessel shape.

Next, the cell cluster arranges itself into a new shape. The old shape of a cell colony allowed for entrainment, proximity, and coordinated directional movement. The vessel shape offered a new strategy for the capture and processing of food.

The cell colony, the cluster of protozoan cells, is followed by simple multi-celled creatures called sponges in which cells have specialized roles. One step further in complexity brings us to cnidarians (coelenterates), radially symmetrical creatures planted on a pond, or lake or ocean floor. These include the hydra, the sea anemone, or the free-floating jellyfish. These creatures are basically invaginated spheres—spheres that are dimpled and turned partly outside in. We use the descriptive term Vessel for such creatures. Cnidarians are primarily a gut body; they feed by catching particles that float by, using flagella to bring them into the gut for digestion. Capturing food, digesting it, and releasing unwanted portions constitute the major events of these creatures' lives.

The vessel body is also used to represent the original emergence of a gut nervous system, a neural net that spans the walls of the hydra. The association of gut tissue, and a neural net within, is a convenient analogy to the neural network of the human gut, dubbed the enteric brain by current researchers.[1] Gut feelings now have some scientific credibility. [2,3]

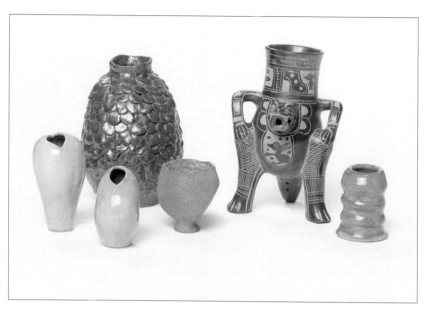

Fig.6.4. *Shown above are various ceramic vessels, a form created throughout history.*
(Photograph by John Hession.)

Exercise:
EMBODYING THE VESSEL — VESSEL BREATH

Look at the pictures of the hydra. It is a vessel, like a bowl or a cup, with an opening at the top. This shape permeates human history in endless varieties of form and function. It resides in our unconscious as a symbol of woman or matrix.

The hydra is planted on the lake floor with flagella extending beyond its top, waving in the watery currents.

Begin your exploration of Vessel by sitting on the floor or a chair. You can also be on hands and knees, or lie down. Open your mouth gently and begin to make an audible breath, a sound like a soft "haw" from the bottom of the throat. Explore opening the mouth wide like the top of the hydra and appreciate the hollow volume of the mouth and throat cavity, using the sensation of breath to

locate perception within them. Or open the mouth a tiny bit and build the space of mouth and gut tube so there may be a slow relaxation from the inside out. Use the breath and the sense of breathing the volume of your body. Imagine a hollow gut within your body from top to bottom. Imagine breathing in the sea to create a hollowing process until you reach the bottom of your trunk—the pelvic floor. You might imagine tasting the sea as you create space inside you.

Breathe into the theatre of this exploration slowly and gently. Sometimes just the act of bringing attention to the mouth and gut, beginning the opening process is enough for a first time. You may access this process in different ways. You may need to explore the gut gradually, in stages. Try to dilate the sense of your hollow gut, using whatever aspects of the metaphor are helpful. Over time, more of your gut may begin to speak to you and become accessible.

Explore becoming a simple vessel, "disappearing" your spine and limbs. Experiment with the amount of curve in the neck to find the easiest posture for feeling the neck of the vessel. What is the felt sense of the gut body? Let your effort and intention be given a chance to sink in. Take a drink of water; notice swallowing, smelling, tasting, and sensing temperature, from a place of Vessel awareness. How is this feeling similar to or different from Cell or Cell Colony?

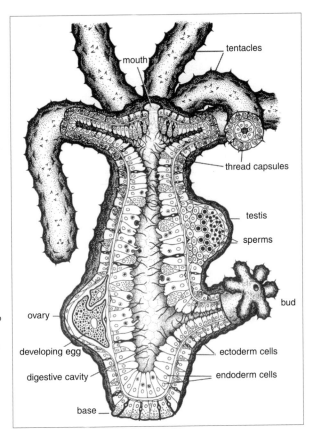

Fig.6.5. *Shown at right: A hydra, in cutaway view to reveal its shape and two layers of cells.* (Reproduced with permission from Buchsbaum, R., Buchsbaum, M., Pearse, V., and Pearse, J., *Animals Without Backbones: An Introduction to the Invertebrates,* Third Edition. Chicago: University of Chicago Press, 1987, p. 89.)

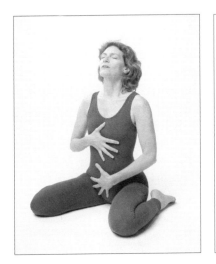 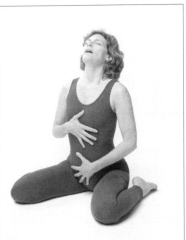 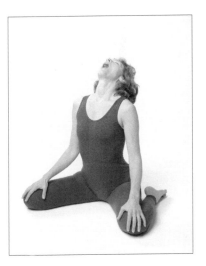

Figs. 6.6a,b,c. *Feeling into the gut body using breath, sound, movement, and imagination to embody Vessel.* (Photographs by John Hession.)

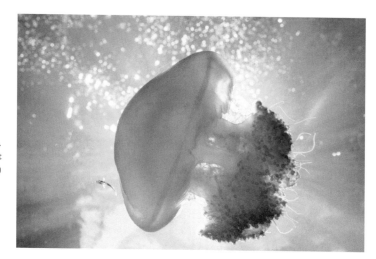

Fig.6.7. *Jellyfish, a cnidarian.*
(Reproduced with permission from Chris Newbert
and Brigitte Wilms/Minden Pictures.)

Experiment with moving like the hydra, planted in one spot and moved by the surrounding ocean current, or like the jellyfish, floating and pulsating. Allow simple wave motions to move you on the floor, or feel the subtle internal wave motion.

NOTES FOR TEACHERS AND BODY THERAPISTS ON VESSEL

The gut body has particular significance in our culture of gut denial. Habitual contraction of the abdominal wall is a common source of strain in bodies. Many people have been encouraged to hold their belly walls tight. This effort has led to an epidemic of flattened lumbar spines and locked pelvises, as well as bottled-up emotions.

The vessel breath allows the abdominal contents to be in a more natural state. We want to shift the context from familiar associations of "stomach" or "belly," to remove a primary source of strain and inhibition, and initiate empowering movement and flow in the body.

Learning to "let go" of the abdominal muscles is a difficult and frustrating task for many people. The vessel breath and the subsequent vessel movement are tools that allow the body to self-organize at a gut level. Opening the mouth wide and making the audible breath contradicts inhibition in facial expression, specifically in the lips and teeth and tongue. These are the openings of the gut, and they can affect or be deeply affected by explorations of the gut.

Finding and amplifying the felt sense of calm and of relaxation in the digestive organs and abdominal tissue helps to modify autonomic balance. The mechanism for this is not scientifically clear. Why should what we feel in the belly change our sympathetic and parasympathetic balance?

Life's challenges often rob us of the simple act of feeling content. A simple noticing of contentment in our belly may help restore health and well-being. Negative images of our belly and constant external sensory stimuli are just factors that turn off our ability to feel simple belly contentment.

A content belly, a healthy gut, has organic, rhythmic intelligence and intrinsic wave-like motions. There is natural therapeutic value in learning to sense the waves of movement that occur within us. This movement is occurring all the time. It is the product of what science calls vegetative consciousness, the action of brain stem and local intelligence of the tissue itself.

Why are we calmed when we sense this movement? Empirical evidence says that people can calm themselves using visualization and noticing their breath. When we sense the wave motion inside us, are we merely helping ourselves to let go of stressful thoughts and patterns, or is there a more direct link? Does stimulating gut body movement speak to the nervous system through other pathways, more directly?

What we sense in our abdomen is not limited to contentment. We may sense a whole spectrum of feelings. Before we call them feelings, we may notice a myriad of sensations—movements, sounds, pulsations. As we feel deeply the kaleidoscope of sensory phenomena that occur in the gut body, we may also begin to notice shifts of sensation in other parts of our body. These shifts can indicate significant autonomic adjustments, such things as changes in the circulation of blood, or heart and respiratory rate. There may also be unusual adjustments to tonic function.

Consider this account by a movement student. It speaks to perception, the shift of perception that comes from using movement, imagination, and breath:

"I had spent about twenty minutes investigating the digestive tube through breath. I explored the widening of my jaw to its limits and beyond. I imagined the tube widening all the way down into the bottom of my gut. I allowed the bottom of my gut to expand and settle and expand further and settle more. I could call the way I felt a 'trance state' and yet, if there had been an emergency, my body would have snapped out of it instantly. I came, after some time, to rest with my belly on the floor. I felt melted into the floor in a pleasurable

ecstasy I could not have previously imagined. I felt the other participants breathing and softly moving nearby. My body was the whole room and everyone in it. I felt a sense of rest unlike any I had felt before. My body was truly lying down and letting itself drop. Astonishment, relief, and gratitude were the thoughts that lightly occurred. But thoughts were dwarfed by the felt sense of rest and expansion. And I heard the teacher announce that it was time to create slow transition. I tried to move, gently. And as long as my efforts were gentle, I was amazed to find that I felt too heavy to move. My back muscles, my muscles of arousal to gravity, were asleep! I struggled amusedly for some time, arising slightly and falling back to Earth. I laughed quietly and a little bit self-consciously at my plight. The reins of tonic function had let go. My upright character was temporarily disconnected."

Some people might not identify with this story. Indeed, not being able to budge from bed sells coffee. However, there are those for whom difficulty rising from bed is not the problem. The problem is finding a way to relax and recover from a perpetual life of exhausting activity and worry. Movement study seems to allow the body to balance its autonomic system whichever side it is tuned to.

Restoring our ability to feel doesn't deliver us to an ideal primitive state. We are doing something different than returning to our babyhood or returning to some primitive experience. We want to couple our capacity to observe and think abstractly with the basic intelligence of our gut tissue.

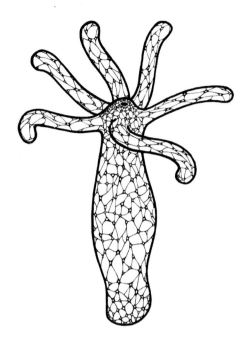

Fig.6.8. *Diagram indicating the nerve net throughout the outer cell layer of the hydra.* (Reproduced with permission from Buchsbaum, R., Buchsbaum, M., Pearse, V., and Pearse, J., *Animals Without Backbones: An Introduction to the Invertebrates,* Third Edition. Chicago: University of Chicago Press, 1987, p. 100.)

TISSUE DIFFERENTIATION

An important lesson in this chapter is about tissue differentiation. We play in the imagination with a creature that has two distinct types of tissue: nerve tissue in the form of a neural net or ectoderm, and gut tissue that is inner tissue or endoderm. Two functions have been separated into essentially two layers of tissue: one for sensing and protection, and one for digesting.

Another lesson is about form. The cell and cell colony represent spherical forms. Cnidarians, vessel creatures, are radially symmetrical forms. The body of the vessel creature is arranged around its hollowness, its chamber. The chamber has within it an implied axis. Although there is no tissue defining the axis, the shape implies the center point around which all the tissue is radially symmetrical. We have played with two of the basic life forms on Earth. We will visit a third form in the next chapter.

We have established ourselves, with a boundary and gut, found awareness of space and weight. Where does our story go next? Each innovation in evolution brings new complexity. We can experience each stage of complexity in our bodies. As we embody each new creature, we invite the reader to solve an analogous human challenge.

Do we need this kind of challenge? Some may ask, why do people need this kind of work? If humans are a result of 2 billion years of innovation, why is there value in rolling around on the floor and making primitive sounds? Humans have become chair-dwelling, car-riding, machine-operating, industrialized beings—largely divorced from the natural rhythms and activities of nature in which we evolved. At the same time, human beings are engaged in many bold evolutionary experiments. We make self-improvements by extending life span, and by, for example, examining the mental and emotional health of each other. All this is brand new, in an evolutionary time scale.

As practitioners of movement, we see many people looking for comfort with the ancient and the modern in their bodies, with the need to adapt and change. Playing in the metaphors of evolution can help us open our perception and find links between the ancient and the new.

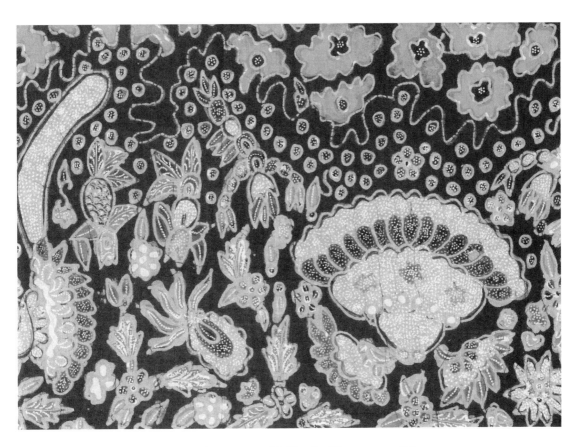

Fig.6.9. *"Marine Life" (detail of Javanese textile).*

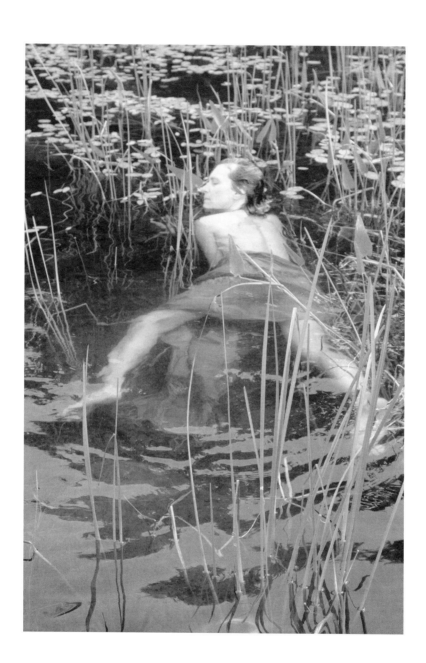

CHAPTER 7

Mobility—
the Gut Body Gains an Axis

The hydra fastens itself to the bottom of a lake. Food comes to it. Its flagella help snare the food. The gut body is vegetative, passive, rooted—in touch with the ground. We visit the vessel to explore a sense of ground, of the "down" direction.

Our story is going to make a jump, a creative leap that strikes a contrast with the simplicity and groundedness of Vessel. All the creatures that follow embody this next step. Our human form and behavior have this step built in from the moment of conception.

The next step is to find direction in space, and to move forward—to pop out of groundedness and penetrate space with our intention and our physical body. What does this mean for sensate exploration? What does this do to the shape and organization of the body? Popping out of groundedness and moving forward in space define dimensions of physical space—left/right, up/down, front/back. By defining these dimensions, form differentiates and organizes—bilateral symmetry emerges. Life has a new model. Every subsequent life form depends on this innovation, in the same way that technology depends on electricity.

The innovation shifts from an organism that is radially symmetrical to an organism with an axis. By an axis we mean a line around which a shape is built. We find a tube-shaped creature that has a front and back end, a top and bottom, and two sides. This new shape is said to have *bilateral symmetry.*

POPPING OUT

Can you remember a time when you leapt forth, energetically, psychologically, or physically? See what comes to mind. Track what you sense in your body as you remember popping out. Then notice the moments before popping, before the idea of popping entered your system. What happened to trigger the pop? Can you tell? Or notice the moment of popping itself.

What do you remember? You may wish to move the sense of what you remember, to experiment with your pop. What does the body do to pop?

Here are other people's experiences of popping:

A woman reports: *"I am lying in bed, dozing and also waiting for the alarm to buzz. I'm thinking about the day to come, the meeting with so and so. … I'm also feeling heavy, appreciating the warm body next to mine, the quiet of the early morning. All of a sudden, I remember the laundry that has to be dry so I can wear the clothes. I find my body leaping out of the bed. I imagine damp, sour turtlenecks and underwear mashed against the tub of the washing machine.*

The picture of the clothes is coupled with the picture of a clock and a picture of me driving to work and a picture of those clothes on my body with damp spots. The heaviness of my body is suddenly gone.

"As I moved this experience in class, I was curious about the shape sense of my body, before, during, and after the pop as you call it. I drew these shapes. The shape before popping is a purple and brown pancake; the shape during popping is a yellow lightning bolt with stars floating around it. The shape moments after the pop is a blue-white oblong with limbs radiating out of it; the oblong leans forward."

Another woman reports: *"I was at a dinner party listening to several men talk housebuilding— I was thinking to myself, how boring. One of them, across the table, started talking about how he likes working with concrete because he can build houses like the ones he remembers he stayed in as a child on the Greek islands. Then I thought, oh cool, I was in Greece a few years ago. Those island houses are really beautiful! I felt myself get upright in my chair and start babbling about the Greek island houses and that I knew just what he meant.*

"I felt a little bit embarrassed afterward. I couldn't help myself and I know it was not very cool to get so suddenly excited. No one seemed to mind, but the popping thing you are talking about makes sense. I was sitting listening, judging, restless in my chair. When the idea of the Greek islands came up, I felt my energy fly across the table toward the guy who was talking about it.

"I think the pop came in my chest, like a little explosion. My toes curled a little bit and pressed down against the floor."

Popping out means accelerating in the direction of something that excites us. It may involve a gross shift in body shape or movement, or an energetic or perceptual shift. However, all popping out involves a direction in space. See if you can appreciate how the vessel is different from something that can pop out.

The vessel is rooted in one place. Its flagella wave in the currents of the surrounding water. Food falls by chance into the vessel. There is no apparent action that the vessel can take to influence its fate. By contrast, popping out is a leap of possibility! The new possibility is the surge of energy and the acceleration that enables a creature to move in a direction.

What happened in our evolutionary story so that creatures could pop out? Early cells did have flagella (tails) that could push them forward. How did multi-celled creatures begin to move?

Evolutionary biologists found one possible solution when they considered the step from stationary filter feeder to mobile filter feeder.

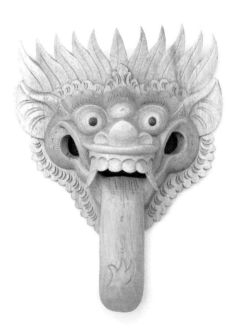

Fig. 7.2. *Balinese wood carving of Barong, protector of mankind.*

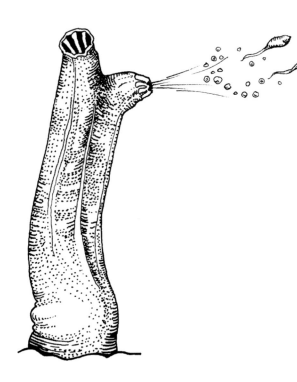

Fig. 7.3. *Diagram of tunicate filter feeder, with larvae freely swimming. Scientists speculate that some larvae may have remained swimmers in their adult form.* (Drawing by Susan Kress Hamilton.)

THE CHORDATE—THE LANCELET

The lancelet is a primitive chordate. The step to being a chordate is a dramatic change from the simple vessel. The lancelet has an axis. It swims by using the movement of its tail and fin. It is a filter feeder that can pursue what it feeds on, can go forth into space. In doing this, it becomes a tube-like body shape. First there is a gut vessel, but now it is contained within an overall tube-like body plan. The gut elongates and becomes tubular in shape. This new mobile form expresses other features as well. The lancelet has a front end and a back end, a top and a bottom, and a right and left—all this follows from moving out, popping out, into space. The body also acquires a notochord, a primitive stiffening rod that allows the musculature of this tube body to focus the force of its movements into a wave form that pushes it forward in the water. In addition to the nerve net in the gut, the new body has a dorsal nerve cord positioned above the notochord.

Feel the shift that took place in form and movement from the vessel creature to the primitive swimming tube.

Feel yourself as a radially symmetrical creature—the vessel. Your sense of body is round and connected to the ground. What does the space around you feel like?

Next, imagine something enticing, something that inspires you to pop out. Notice the shift in your body's felt sense. How does your body prepare? What happens to your sense of shape? What happens to your sense of space?

They theorize that the filter feeding tunicate (a form of complex vessel creature) gave rise to chordates, the first creatures with a primitive backbone. Look at the illustration of the tunicate. The larval (immature) form of the tunicate is a mobile tadpole. As the tunicate matures, it loses its mobility and settles down in one spot, anchored to the floor of the ocean. Evolutionary biologists asked the question, what if one of these larval tadpole creatures never grew up? What if, instead of maturing into the rooted tunicate adult, one of the tadpoles remained mobile? What would evolve is a creature with an axis from a creature that was radially symmetrical.

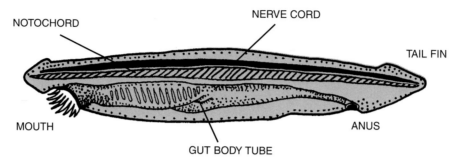

NOTOCHORD

NERVE CORD

TAIL FIN

MOUTH

ANUS

GUT BODY TUBE

Fig. 7.4. *Diagram of a lancelet, a chordate filter feeder, free swimming but more primitive than fish.* (Drawing by Susan Kress Hamilton.)

Creatures built around an axis express their movement in their shape. The direction of their movement is defined by how the head is pointed. An arrow can be used to represent the vector of movement, and in a creature the head is the point of that arrow. Where the head points, the creature goes—the axis of the body follows the head. Form follows the function of the creature.

Exercise:
FINDING AN AXIS—
ESTABLISHING THE TUBE BODY

To feel the development of an axis, we start by feeling our head.

Place the top of your head on the floor or wall. Begin to roll and pour the container of the skull. Explore the rhythm and pace that is the most interesting and feel the variety of sensations produced by rolling the surfaces of the skull. Pause periodically and notice the arising of impulse to move, the impulse to explore sensation in the skull.

In a seated position, notice the skull in space. Can you sense the surface of your head as it meets the air? Play with tiny movements of the skull in space and feel the direction through the top of your head.

Exercise:
CONE HEAD EXERCISE

To find your cone head, close your eyes, and imagine a conical projection growing out of the top of your head. This exercise should be done gradually, with careful attention to changes in extended proprioception. Slowly grow the cone until you feel it to be about thirteen inches tall. (By slowly we suggest you take a few seconds to add each inch of height to your imagined cone head.) Move the tip of the cone head in space in a small circle. Feel the extended sense of body into the space above your head. Initiate micro-movements. Imagine that you greet or touch another with your cone head tip.

Relax into the deep fold, the position of feeling the cell. Establish a sense of omni-directional awareness. Feel your skin and your sense of contents. Begin to arouse a feeling of the cone head, a sense that one's head can explore space and penetrate space. Let the head carry you into space, making tiny exploratory wave motions with the head. Then let the wave motion travel down the axis of your spine. Imagine, instead of a spine, your axis is softer cartilaginous tissue. This enables you to wiggle freely as you explore moving out into space. Wiggling forward on the floor establishes the creature body that is axial, that has a front end and a tail, a top and bottom, and a right and left side. Return to feeling the vessel shape of your body, and reestablish your axis with the point of your head. What are the feeling qualities of these two body attitudes?

Having an axis, you are capable of directing yourself toward or away from an object. As you wiggle on the floor, notice how your eyes and head organize your direction. Start with a sense of your contents, your grounded vessel body; then let your eyes orient to an object. What happens to your sense of body and space? Notice how having an axis is absolutely necessary for efficient movement. If you had a gelatinous body with no stiffening rod, your movement would be more random—you would have trouble reaching your goal quickly. Remember the place of all possibilities in being Cell? Now there is only one possibility being chosen and you pop in that direction.

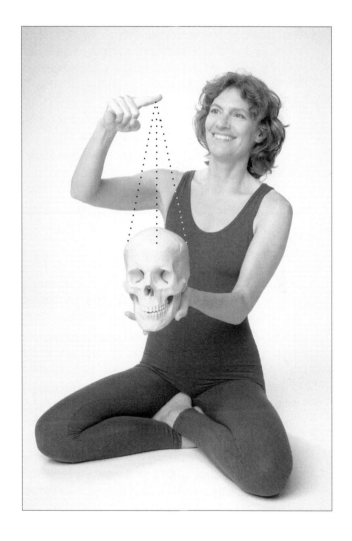

Fig. 7.5 at right. *Imagine growing a conical projection out of the top of your head. How does this change your sense of axis, of space, and of movement?* (Photograph by John Hession.)

NOTES FOR TEACHERS AND BODY THERAPISTS ON EXPLORING THE AXIS LINE

The transition from tunicate to chordate offers us awareness of what it means to be formed around an axis. Chordates, creatures like fish, reptiles, and mammals including humans—all have a central axis or line. Feeling the potency of this line is one of the central points of Ida Rolf's work. It is also found in many of the body disciplines and spiritual traditions that are woven into human history.

Yoga and Zen Buddhism are just two of the human traditions that point to the value of feeling a "line." These traditions use the concept of line to orient to gravity, upright, with the bottom end of the spine pointing toward the ground and the top of the head pointed toward the sky. Here we explore the evolutionary step in which the sense of line was first possible.

FEELING OUR LINE

Reconsider the difference between feeling one's internal environment and, orienting to space, what is outside one's body. Feeling a linear direction is one of the possibilities when we orient to space. Sensing a direction in space affects our body movement and consequently our body shape. Orientation leads to a shape defined by the directionality of perception. You see forward in a straight line and your shape becomes a straight line. The stronger you orient, the more your body extends its line. The less you orient in a direction, the less your body exhibits a sense of linear movement.

Can you observe this in moving people? At an airport, mall, or school, can you see how the shape and intention of movement is congruent with the body shape? Observing those with necks and chests pointed forward toward their goal, how does this movement attitude show up in body shape?

How does a strong capacity or tendency to pop out show up in body shape? How does it show up in your own body? Are parts of your body willing to pop forward, to orient, and other parts less willing? These are tricky questions. Bodies change their orienting styles in different contexts.

Orientation lives in our body and shapes our movement. By noticing how orientation initiates, we differentiate our perception of ourselves and of others.

The early axial body—in this case, the lancelet—is the foundation for anatomical organization in fish, amphibians, reptiles, and mammals. Students of anatomy and body therapy can appreciate how organs, muscles, and bones organize around a line. The transition from vessel shape to tube shape helps us imagine how the impulse to move forward into space determined the blueprint for all the complex creatures to follow.

There are now three categories of tissue. The lancelet has a gut and a nervous system. The cartilaginous stiffening rod, or notochord, represents a third tissue that provides support. The axial shape brings with it a way to hold its shape and helps with locomotion. This is mesoderm. Muscles, bones, and fascia belong to this category. The form of our bodies begins to emerge.

We appreciate the power of the line to determine and hold form. We appreciate the power of orientation to shape movement and body-form. The power of orientation helps us understand why movement study pioneers taught their students to understand and use this perceptual force for performance, for healing, and as a chance to awaken consciousness. The evolutionary story illustrates how the impulse to move in a direction brought with it enormous consequences.

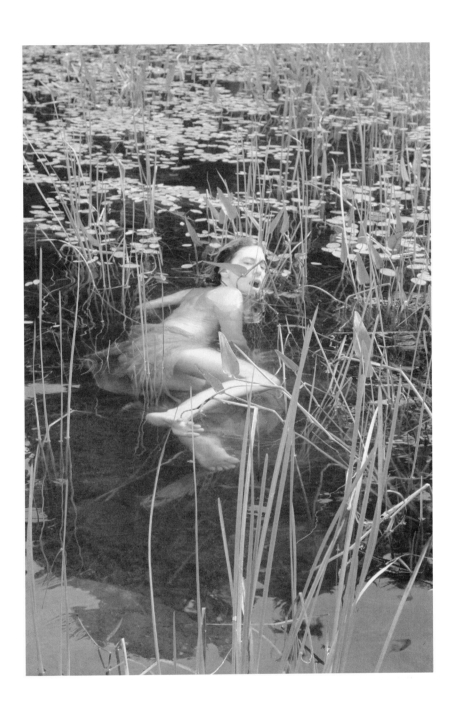

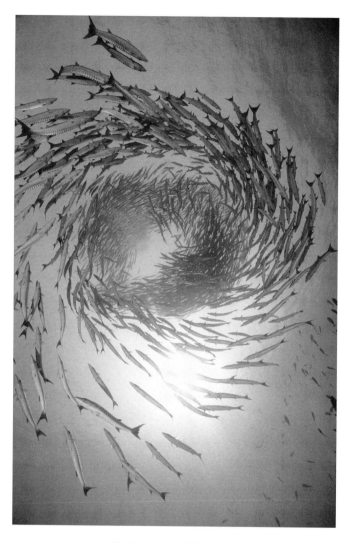

Fig. 8.1. *School of barracuda.*
(Reproduced with permission from Chris Newbert/Minden Pictures.)

Chapter 8

Lateral Line – the Fish Body

Bilateral symmetry is formalized in the fish. The fish has a head, tail, spine, ribs, and fins. The fish shows us a body with features found in amphibians, reptiles, and mammals, including human mammals—but without limbs. The side-to-side swishes of a fish move it along in the water. This side-bending appears in all the later creatures as lateral flexion of the spine. The fish has a lateral line that is pressure sensitive and allows the fish to sense what is beside it.

LATERAL LINE

Lateral Line is a concept used by biologists and practitioners of Structural Integration. Ida Rolf used the lateral line of the human body to show how different bodies have different organization in gravity. Probably there are many other specialized uses of the term Lateral Line. We want to ground this concept as something to feel in your body.

To help orient our human body to the perspective of the fish, search your memory for an experience of having a lateral line. Think about the sides of your body, as opposed to your front and back surfaces. Feel into the sense of your sides. When has this orientation been relevant?

Have you stood shoulder to shoulder in a line? Have you lain side by side with someone? Do you sleep on your side—and have you ever not been able to sleep on one side or the other? Have you been in competition, a race, or some competitive event where your competitor is to one side or the other? Has your pet walked by your side? Have you walked in a parade with one person or more beside you? Have you danced in a circle holding hands with those beside you? Have you stood in an elevator with unfamiliar people on either side of you?

Find some experience where you notice the world through the side of your body. Bring the memory into sensation. What is it like to notice your awareness through the side of your body?

Your awareness may be quite subtle or it may be strong and surprising. Just notice it and make note of your discovery. Do you resist this exercise? This may happen if the concept of Lateral Line is new. Noticing your own lateral line may feel abstract at first. Through noticing sensations this may change.

Here are some observations of others:
One person says: *"I remember riding on the train to New York City from Albany. I'd sit down in a seat by the window, and eventually the train was pretty full and someone would ask me if the*

seat next to me was free. I'd say yes and then there would be a new body two inches to my right or left. I'd feel a fuzzy feeling on my side and I would focus on noticing how that space next to me felt. I would imagine I could feel the energy of the person next to me."

A second person reports also being on a train, but a subway train, so he was standing up. The train car was very crowded and as people pressed around him, he found that his sense of personal space was most acute on his left side. He used his elbow to fend off anyone getting too close.

One woman speaks about her experience in dance classes: "I liked sliding sideways, either by myself or in a circle with others. I liked the power feeling of the whole group moving sideways. To be moving with the narrow part of my body was a novel and liberating sensation."

Occasionally the response might be: "This exercise doesn't make a lot of sense to me. I don't see anything different about the side of me, from the front or the back. I am irritated that we were asked to spend time doing this. You can make anything out of anything. What's the point?"

Another person comments: "Have you ever seen the movement of a fish out of water flopping from one side to another?"

Lateral Line, like gravity, is a concept that can, at first, be unsettling. The tendency for the body to self-organize may be relevant to exercises that involve a new word or idea. If someone acknowledges a reaction—annoyance, for example—and then allows his or her body to improvise, exploring the sensations and impulses that arise, there may be a resolution without thinking about it.

LATERAL FLEXION

Our spine bends from side to side in lateral flexion. In a fish, the ribs make a hoop that is long and flattened on the side of its body. For later creatures, this rib shape no longer made sense. In humans we can bend forward and backward. Our ribs are broad and flattened in our front and back surfaces, and narrow on the side. We can still bend to the side, however, while the fish isn't able to bend forward and backward. This allows humans to retain fish movement and to experience it.

Fig. 8.2. *Fish diagram with Lateral Line.*
(Drawing by Susan Kress Hamilton.)

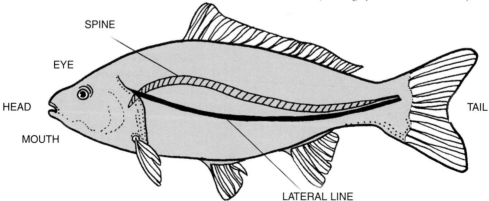

Here are a few exercises that help build a perception of Lateral Line and find the movement of lateral flexion.

First, we use perception to find a sense of the movement.

Lie on your back on a smooth, slippery floor. Enliven your sense of space to the side of your body by feeling the lateral line. Then find a sense of the space that extends away from your lateral line. Begin to bend to one side, imagining that you are bending the space alongside your body. You may bend the space on the convex side by putting a bulge in that space or you may wrap the space within the curve of the concave side. You are relating the sensation of the side of your body to the imagined sense of the space next to it. Let the shape of the space orient your perception. Bend to the opposite side. Sense your lateral line and then build the sense of space before moving. This perceptual process is the beginning of the movement. This is an example of pre-movement. Repeat this several times. Notice your body and register your experience as a baseline for later comparison.

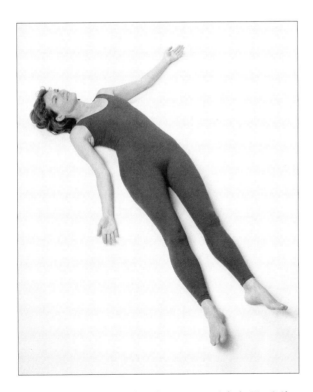

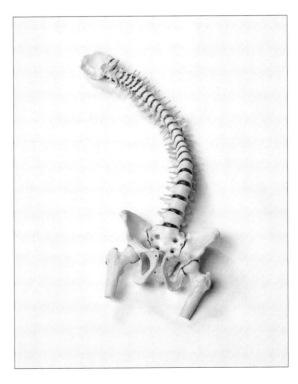

Fig.8.3a on left. *Side-bending the spine in one's body.* Fig. 8.3b on right. *Model of the spine side-bending.* (Photographs by John Hession.)

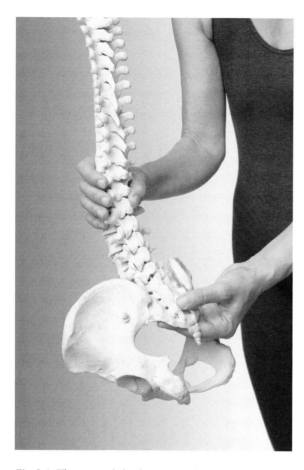

Fig. 8.4. *The spine includes the sacrum and coccyx. The two halves of the pelvis attach to the spine at the sacroiliac joints.* (Photograph by John Hession.)

Reestablish your sense of head, as you did for tube body exploration. Find the sense of skull by rolling and pouring it on a surface, and/or feel the imaginary cone head that extends your axis out the top of your head. Find your axis by reaching forward from the top of your head into space.

The fish has a noticeable tail. When we popped out, the head moved into space first, and the body trailed behind, ending in what we call *Tail*. We need to establish Tail. In the deep fold, locate the lower end of your spine by reaching down and touching it. You will feel the tip end of the spine or close to it. That is the coccyx. The bony mass directly above your coccyx is called the sacrum. Bring your attention to the bottom of your gut body and let the breath touch these tissues. You are breathing into what is called the pelvic floor. Attend to your sense of coccyx and sacrum and feel the breath touching these bony parts as well. See what kinds of sensations and movements the breath provokes in this part of your body.

Now begin to imagine that the tail end of your spine is moving in space. The coccyx is the pointer that aims this movement. The sacrum adds its mass and depth to the movement impulse. Come onto your hands and knees. Follow the movement impulses of your coccyx and sacrum, in space, allowing the tail end of your spine to lead you back into the deep fold.

In the deep fold, notice the top of your head. Slowly extend the cone head pointer into space and explore the movement, playing with small wiggles, undulations, or wave motions. Notice your tail again. Let the tail lead you in wiggles and waves. Imagine a vector from your tail that reaches into the space behind you. Let that guide your movement. Generally, we are not as used to orienting direction with our tail. What is it like to wiggle into space from the head end, and from the tail end? In either direction you define an axis of movement. As you alternate, you grow in an established sense of two directions in the axis.

Staying in the deep fold, breathe into the low back. Invite the breath into one side of the low back. A partner's hand on this area will make it easier to feel and direct the breath. See if it's possible to breathe with a sense that one side of the low back expands and lengthens. After expanding and lengthening one side of the low back with the breath, invite the expansion and lengthening into the other side.

With an established sense of head and tail, breathe into the two halves of the lower back. Come out of the deep fold, slowly turning onto your back.

The beginning of your movement is the perception of head and tail, the head pointer extending beyond the top of the head, the tail pointer extending your tail. Recall the vessel feeling. Allow the gut body to feel its weight and to be soft. Using the newly enlivened feeling of breath in one side of the low back, let the breath lengthen that side and expand into the adjacent space. This is a slow, gentle movement, allowing the sense of breath and building the sense of space. Explore the possibilities for lengthening on both sides, from a sense of breath, a sense of space, a sense of head and tail. Notice whether your gut body can stay heavy and soft. Let the lengthening of one side create the lateral flexion. Initiate the bend to the opposite side through feeling breath and space and head and tail.

Recall the notochord of the lancelet (the cartilaginous stiffening rod) as your axis and feel the power of that axis to reach simultaneously in two directions. Use the sense of notochord to help you feel the side-to-side swish of the fish.

Can you recall your baseline before you established head and tail and before breathing and lengthening the two sides of the low back? See if you can use words to articulate the contrast. What are the qualities of sensation, of movement, of effort, of space in each instance?

Explore your impulses in lateral flexion. You may wish to alternate between large, dynamic sweeps of the spine, and more subtle wiggles or micro-movements. Movement may transport you across the floor or you may stay in one place and notice differentiated sensations of the spine.

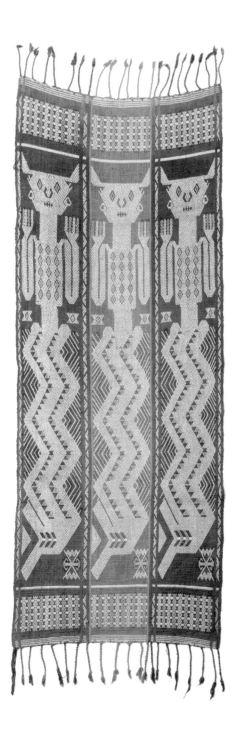

Fig. 8.5. *"Mermen" (Indonesian textile)*.
(Photograph by John Hession.)

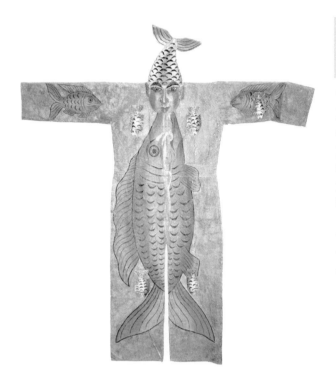

Exercise:
Fish Swish on the Back

This is a partnered exercise. One partner lies on his or her back. The other holds that person's ankles and lifts them, elevating the legs. Slide the person across the floor creating a side-to-side swish. This allows the partner on the floor to feel a passive but dynamic flow of side-to-side movement in the spine.

A solo exploration is to take a walk and sense the lateral flexion in the spine. Switch between the human walk and the exploration of human doing fish movement on the floor.

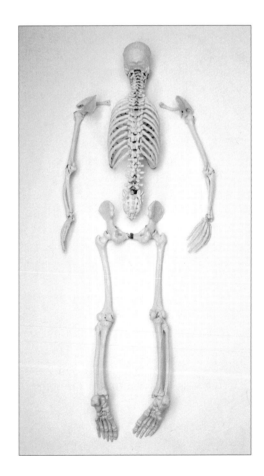

Fig. 8.6. *Fish costume from the Yucatan, Mexico.*

Fig. 8.7. *The fish body plan (head, spine, rib cage, and tail) revealed in this model of the human body by detaching the shoulder and pelvic girdles.* (Photograph by John Hession.)

The human rib cage is joined to the spine in the back and to the sternum in the front. The lowest ribs reach to the waist on the side and the uppermost ribs form the base of the neck.

Although our ribs are shaped differently, we have a similar body plan to the fish. We both have a head-to-tail axis and a rib cage *(see figures 8.7, 8.8, and 8.9.)*

The idea of not having your shoulder girdle and your pelvic girdle may be shocking or disturbing. No pelvis and shoulder blades, no arms or legs, no hands or feet—this predicament doesn't make much sense on land, as a mammal. In movement study the experience may turn out to be different than the idea. In the case of the fish body, we invite you to "disappear" the girdles and visit the fish body as an entry point for differentiated perceptions.

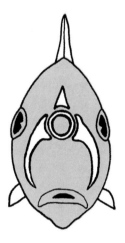

Fig. 8.8. *Fish rib cage compared to human rib cage. Fish ribs are deep front to back and narrow side to side. Human ribs are shallow front to back, relative to width.* (Drawing by Susan Kress Hamilton.)

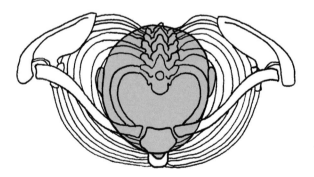

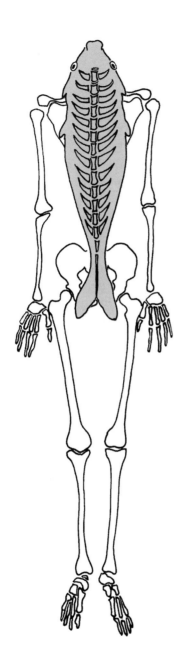

With your fingers, trace the shape of a partner's ribs along the lateral line. (You can also do this on your own.) Trace the shape of the sacrum. Follow its joint with the ilium, or hip bone *(see Figures 10 and 11 a,b).* Use your fingers, or the side of your hand, to "draw" the line from the lateral border of the sacrum to the side of the lower ribs. You are describing the lower end of the fish body. Notice the mass and thickness of the sacrum (independent from the hip bones) as a weight that gives the tail mass and authority for propulsion. Move the lower end of your fish body from side to side with your established sense of tail. Can you grow in the fullness of the lower fish body by moving its contents and outline? Play with this movement until you can initiate with equal clarity from both ends of your spine.

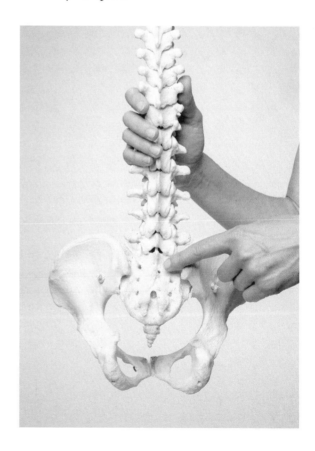

Fig. 8.9 above. *Using fanciful imagination to build the perception of a fish body within our human form.* (Drawing by Susan Kress Hamilton.)

Fig. 8.10 right. *Feel through the soft tissue covering the sacrum and imagine you can trace the sacroiliac joint.* (Photograph by John Hession.)

With your fingers, trace the ribs higher, along the lateral line, until you bump into the arm pit. Allow this arm to rise over the head and the shoulder blade to shift back as far as it can comfortably go. Now continue to trace the ribs, finding them in the sensitive tissue under the arm. As you trace the ribs, give your partner—or yourself, if working alone—adequate time to grow in the sense of having ribs here. Then trace the base of the neck into the space behind the clavicle. Using an audible breath can help mobilize the upper ribs to swing more easily. Although the finger reaching up from the underarm and the finger reaching down from the area behind the clavicle won't meet, the distance may be traveled in your imagination, and you can sense the contour of the upper ribs. Can you feel the outline of your fish body as

separate from the shoulder? Sense the streamlined shape that a fish has, with no shoulders or pelvis. Breathe through your mouth, moving breath into the sides of the ribs, and following the breath up to the side of the neck.

Lie on your back and roll the rib cage on the floor. Let the shoulder girdle move aside so the upper ribs can meet the floor. Embody the weight and curve of the upper ribs. Wiggle the head and tail, establishing the axis of the body. Feel the left and right sides, and feel the dorsal (back) surface on the floor. Then roll onto the ventral (front) surface—feeling the side-to-side motion of lateral flexion in each position and play with swishing like a fish. Explore lateral elongation and lateral undulations of the head, ribs, and spine—the fish body.

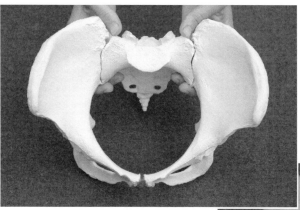

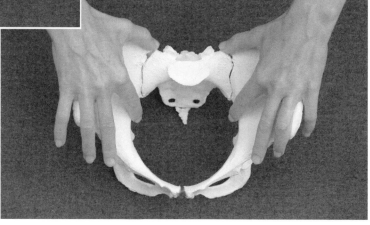

Figs. 8.11a,b.
Showing the sacrum's depth at right and width above.

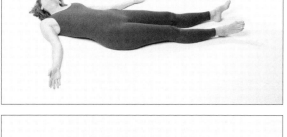

This exercise is best seen demonstrated, but you can get some sense of it from the illustrations. Like all new coordination, it follows from allowing new perception. If you have investigated fish body movement with breath and space, you may have the happy accident of a fish spiral.

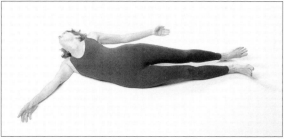

Lie on your back and find out what your body does to roll over onto your front without using your arms and legs.

Notice the side you rolled on. What happened? Where did the movement start? How did it change shape?

Now try this. First, feel the breath expand and lengthen one side of your fish body; let that side open to the space and lengthen in two directions. Orient your eyes to an object on that side and allow your head to follow. See if your fish body is able to lengthen so far that the head movement initiates a rolling over.

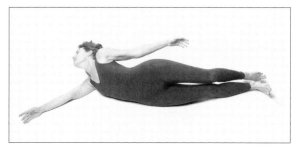

If this is difficult, refresh your perception of head and tail into space so your axis is clear. A clear axis and a clear lengthening response on one side will allow your body to roll over from deep core muscles in a surprising way.

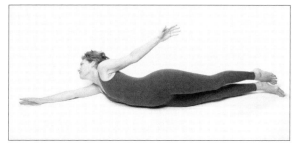

Figs. 8.12a,b,c,d,e. *The fish spiral sequence.*
(Photographs by John Hession.)

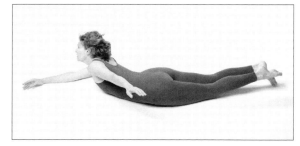

NOTES FOR TEACHERS AND BODY THERAPISTS ON FISH BODY

Sensing our fish body, we establish our axis as having two directions. The sense of two directions in one's axis is a pre-movement, an idea that shows up in many traditions. Yoga, dance, martial arts, and modern movement study, especially as articulated by Ida Rolf, all incorporate the sense of two directions in the vertical line. It is ironic that we use the fish to explore our human axis and gravity response. Fish live in a watery environment where gravity is less noticeable. Yet the body plan with a head and tail and bilaterally symmetric organization is the basis for our human body. Fish are one of the first creatures in which this plan appears.

In the human body we are broad on the front and back rather than the sides; we have limbs and girdles, and our spine bends in additional dimensions. By visiting the fish body we notice our lateral line and learn to perceive through this novel field of awareness. This perception is a portal that unlocks habitual patterns of movement.

Exploration of lateral flexion is an opportunity to improve spinal movement—that is, to change from co-contracted movement to movement in which there is flow. As Ida Rolf put it, "[when] flexors flex, extensors extend."[1] Movement begins by a release of the antagonist rather than engagement of the agonist. It is as if you were able to release your brake pedal and feel your car move before applying the accelerator. A benefit of fish body lateral flexion is the perception that the spine can move without unnecessary compression. The spine can bend with a sense of pleasure and very little effort.

The exercise Fish Body—Disappearing the Girdles allows us to start over in our relationship to our limbs. We may appreciate a sense of freedom from our habitual patterns of discomfort. It is a starting point for untangling shoulder and hip girdle pathologies.

Fish Spiral takes lateral flexion, initiated by lengthening, and turns it into a spinal rotation. Fish aren't able to rotate in this way, at least on land. However, our human body can do rotation, as can sea mammals such as dolphins or whales. Fish Spiral is about rotating without limbs and without compression.

Fish Body illustrates an aspect of the spinal engine theory advanced by Serge Gracovetsky.[2] He showed how the fish body motion is the basic locomotive force in human beings. The side-to-side bending of the spine leads to rotation and counter-rotation of the trunk and pelvis, and by so doing drives the body in walking. Through working with a patient born without legs, Gracovetsky showed that the walking motion is the same whether or not one has legs. Gracovetsky pointed out that any curved but flexible rod, if bent sideways, will rotate.

In the Fish Body exercises it is possible to differentiate the side-bending movement from rotational movement. This process may precipitate improvements in coordination. Diagnosis and treatment of spinal dysfunction derives from feeling the associated side bend and rotational components of spinal segments, and then correcting segments that are rotating improperly.

Movement work claims that maintaining a healthy spine, and even correcting the spine, are possible by differentiating perception and thus improving coordination. In other words, lying down on the floor and feeling lateral flexion, then using breath and imagination to shift the experience of this motion, can and does lead to improved coordination. Taking the time to prepare the movement enables new perceptual details of body and space. As one's perception grows and becomes more finely differentiated, an improvement of function takes place.

By improvement of function we mean less effort is employed by the mover. Brakes are released before the gas pedal is applied. The movement looks and feels more pleasing, more fluid, more graceful, less forced. In addition, close observation will reveal the movement has more complexity. Tiny sub-parts of muscles operate rather than large blocks of muscles.

An improvement of function may follow a lessening of musculoskeletal complaints.

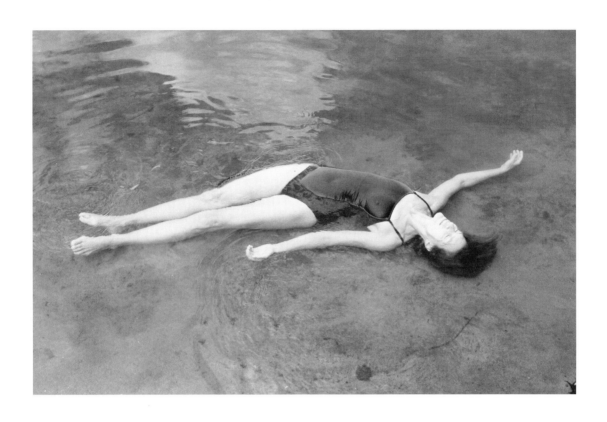

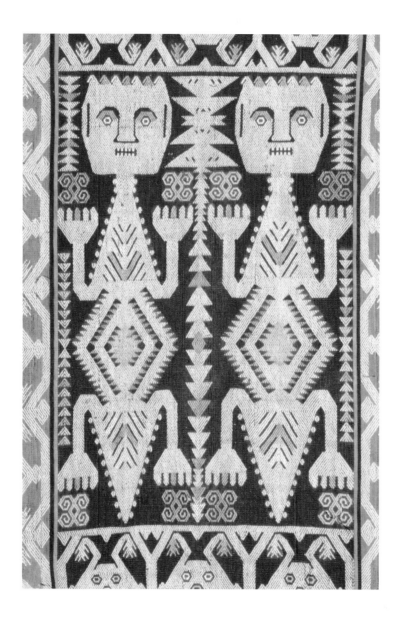

Fig. 9.1. "Reptile Men" (detail of Indonesian textile).

CHAPTER 9

Amphibian and Reptile— Acquiring Girdles

The movement of life from sea to land inspired several body changes. As the watery environment was partly or wholly replaced with shallow water, mud, and land, fins became lobed and fish acquired shoulders and limbs to navigate the transition zones between land and water. The fossil record leaves a gap between fish with limb-like fins, and the first true tetrapods (vertebrates with two pairs of limbs). These first land-based amphibians had weight-bearing limbs and articulated hips and shoulders. Lateral flexion was still the main locomotive strategy, creating a side-to-side wave motion from the head to the tip of the tail.

As amphibians, and then reptiles, moved onto solid ground, gravity became a new factor. Limbs had to lift the trunk off the ground and with this force, the spine had to flex in new ways. To cross over land, the trunk had to bend up and down. We call this movement of the spine *sagittal flexion*— bending forward and backward. Now obstacles could be crossed or avoided.

GRAVITY

Imagine you are a fish and the water around you starts to dry up. Moving over dry land you experience weight differently than in water. Consider gravity, having weight. What does having weight mean to you? What does the concept of living in a gravitational field evoke?

What comes to mind? Find a gesture, a movement, or a series of movements to express your interpretation. Find a movement that captures the felt sense of your internal story, or follow the spontaneous flow of movement that comes from your interpretation. Note what you found out.

Consider these stories:
One man remembers his fantasies about being a giant. As a giant his weight is enormous. Each footstep crunches the ground beneath his giant boots, making places for pools of water to form. He moves as a giant, slowly, savoring the power and mass of largeness. He reenacts the notion that comes to him, that "the bigger they come, the harder they fall," in which he is caught off balance and he crashes to the floor, bouncing repeatedly against the floor.

A woman remembers being thirteen, having developed faster than some of the other girls in her eighth grade class. She feels big, while being really just a healthy girl. The weight of her body feels like it sticks out and is noticeable to everyone. She is conscious of trying to hide her breasts and tucking her belly and buttocks in with her muscles. Now, at age 34, she thinks about how she has learned to relax these restrictions, still being about average in weight, but allowing herself the permission to take up space and have weight on the Earth. In movement, she rehearses the former image of her internal teenager trying to be smaller, and makes leaps through the studio feeling her body's willingness to drop and fly up.

An 84-year-old psychoanalyst is undergoing a Structural Integration series. After his session, he feels a sense of exuberance and goes to the lake for a short swim. As he comes out of the water, the sense of his body having weight is dramatic. His flesh feels substantial; his bones feel dense. He feels alive, noticing freshly the sense of gravity on his human frame. He walks up the hill, lumbering and swinging his arms and shoulders broadly, saying the words, "All right, OK, all right." Each "OK" and "all right" has a joyous ring to it. He also remarks that, recovering his sense of weight and mass, especially in his legs, feels like a reversal of what aging is doing to his perception.

ARTICULATED GIRDLES— SHOULDER AND PELVIC

To appreciate our change in form from fish to amphibian, ask yourself what stories you hold about girdles and limbs.

The words *girdles* and *limbs* will evoke meaning. Try not to judge your self-observations as good or bad, boring or exotic. Notice what they are and let your body's response in movement be the mirror, rather than your evaluative thoughts.

When you hear the terms *shoulder girdle* and *pelvic girdle*, where does your mind go? Does one girdle or limb call you more than another? Do you have a story involving one or more limbs? Note the story and then notice the sensations and impulses in that place in the body. Let them guide you in movement. If no story or association comes to mind, let the invitation to movement be a mystery. Let the notion of girdles guide you unconsciously.

What did you find out about girdles, arms, legs, or just your movement?

Consider these other perspectives:

A woman, age 47, reports: *"After doing the Fish Body exercise, for the first time I realized that my body complaints come from where my girdles join to my Fish Body. Fish Body is a handy way to talk about the trunk before you add the pelvis and shoulder blades and clavicle. Anyway, the places that always hurt are the places where the pelvis joins my ribs and my sacrum. Doing Fish Body I found that without that extra stuff, my body is pretty happy. In my daily life, if things are particularly bad, I feel the tightness in my butt go down into my leg. Sometimes it tingles. I stretch, but I'm beginning to think that stretching may be more helpful if I start to think about the bones and which bones are too stuck together."*

"When I moved, I returned to the feeling of wiggling my spine and letting my girdles rest. Every time I started to move my legs, though, I could feel my habitual leg and pelvis movement come back, not as much as usual. It's really a habit to test if it's in pain and to try to find a way out of its tightness. I moved my spine and my gut body and really had no idea how to add the girdles without the habit coming back."

A musician noticed the girdles in a new way, having visited his Fish Body: *"This is pretty big for me, this girdle and limb idea. The nagging issue has been the way my hand is just not showing up for me when I play the viola. I don't have pain. I don't really have numbness. It's tight, but more than that, my fingers are numbing out and can't be depended upon. I need these arms and hands to do my art, which is music. I almost can't even think about it. Fish Body was the first time in months or maybe years that I felt like I was able to not worry about having working arms and hands and I was surprised by that. So, if you ask me what my story about hands and girdles is, I say, 'what* isn't *my story about it?'"*

This man spent some time doing a slow finger dance in the air, while lying on his back. As can often happen during an exploration time, another student paired up with him and they improvised finger movement together, working with the sense of space as well as shapes of movement in their fingers and hands. The man went on to say, *"My hands feel like they need a vacation in movement that isn't about goals or performance. If I just vegged out, that wouldn't really help. I need to let my hands have some fun or what feels like fun."*

How do these examples relate to your explorations of girdles and limbs? The separation of girdles and trunk is a powerful experience. One can discover freedom in parts of the body that often hurt. That's one of the main points of Fish Body. Even when our limbs and girdles work very happily, this exploration can bring a fresh and lively feeling of our appendages. If we have any chronic or traumatic issues, differentiating limbs from Fish Body can help to reintegrate function and feeling.

GROWING THE GIRDLES BY GROWING THE EXTREMITIES

The fossil record shows fish with limb-like fins, and amphibians with fin-like limbs. Some lobe-finned fish have fins with bones that correspond to what we call our humerus, radius, ulna, and carpal bones. When we compare the present-day lobe-finned fish with the fossil record of the earliest known tetrapod amphibian, Ichthyostega, we see differences. The water-dwelling, lobe-finned fish has limb-like fins and the ancient land-dwelling amphibian Ichthyostega has actual legs and feet. The body comparison shows similarities, however, and helps indicate a transitional moment in the evolutionary story. The metaphor of transition from sea dwelling to land dwelling, from swimmer to crawler, helps rebuild our sense of limbs and girdles in our human bodies.

Our human hands and feet perform many complex tasks and functions. They can register a rich and varied stream of sensations and impressions. It is important to feel, consciously, this stream of sensation—growing an enhanced awareness of sensory impression. We explore the origins of limbs, the beginning of life on land, by sensing through our hands and feet.

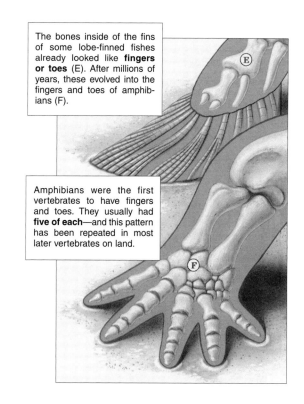

The bones inside of the fins of some lobe-finned fishes already looked like **fingers or toes** (E). After millions of years, these evolved into the fingers and toes of amphibians (F).

Amphibians were the first vertebrates to have fingers and toes. They usually had **five of each**—and this pattern has been repeated in most later vertebrates on land.

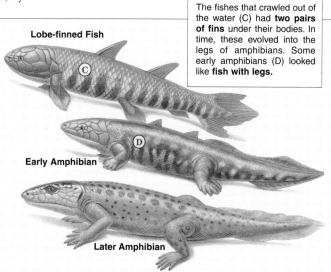

The fishes that crawled out of the water (C) had **two pairs of fins** under their bodies. In time, these evolved into the legs of amphibians. Some early amphibians (D) looked like **fish with legs.**

Lobe-finned Fish

Early Amphibian

Later Amphibian

Figs. 9.2a,b. *The transition from swimmer to crawler expressed in the lobe-finned fish and the early and later amphibian body plans.* (Reproduced with kind permission from John Wexo/Prehistoric Zoobooks.)

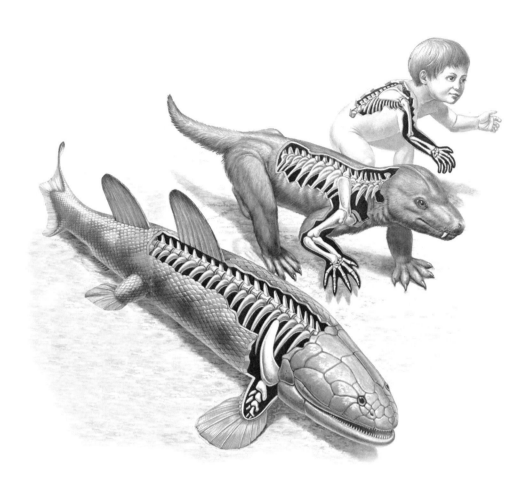

Fig. 9.3. *Comparison of fish, pre-mammal/reptile, and human body plans.* (Reproduced with kind permission from John Wexo/Prehistoric Zoobooks.)

Start by lying on the floor, face-down. Recall the sense of living and moving as a fish. You have a lateral line and move by flexing from side to side.

Bring your hands to the side of your shoulder joint. Your head is turned to the side or is straight, resting on your chin.

Press the skin of your hand against the floor. Feel the texture of the floor. What is the texture like? Can you be curious about the sensations, before thinking about them? Just feel the texture and temperature as it enters the hands.

Now press the floor enough to lift the head and chest a little bit off the floor. Can you still sense in your hands? Often, as our hands begin to act purposefully, our sensing and feeling capacity diminishes. Sometimes refreshing the sense of the fluid body and extending this sense into the finger tips (or toe tips), or imagining a squirting feeling, helps us to maintain sensory awareness in the periphery. Simply slowing the act of pressing the floor to lift the upper body is a chance to integrate sensing and action.

Can you feel the muscles of the shoulder and arm assist the hand in loading? What would it mean to press and lift using only the tips of your fingers? A lobe-finned fish or a frog fish can use the fin strut to navigate coral but doesn't have to bear weight. Coming onto land, the Ichthyostega has a functionally very different limb that bends at a wrist and affords the attachment of stabilizer muscles sufficient to bear the weight of its body. Play between fin-like sensation and limb-like sensation as you raise head and chest off the floor.

Use the vessel breath and gentle wave motion of the gut to find the sense of primitive gut body. Lying supine now, spread the limbs like a starfish. Let the soft motion in the gut travel into one side

of the ribcage, so the motion flows into the shoulder, arm, wrist, and fingers. Do this on both sides. Follow the soft motion from the gut into one side of the pelvis, down into the leg and foot. In connecting all limbs, take the time to establish your center as having depth, not just the belly surface. Follow the sensation, using micro-movement and wave motion from finger tips to gut and back again. Do this with both arms and legs, and then head and tail. Allow yourself to explore the sense of feeling your body as limbs.

In partners, pull gently on each limb. Track the path of sensation from limb to the center of the body. Grow a tangible sense of being all limbs, of having all limbs connect to the center.

Stay with the awareness of limbs sprouting from rib cage and spine, connecting to the center of the body. Now sweep the limbs back and forth on the floor. Turn onto your belly. Quiet the limbs and notice the entire ventral surface of your body resting on the ground. Take time to let the gut body drop fully into the ground; notice support

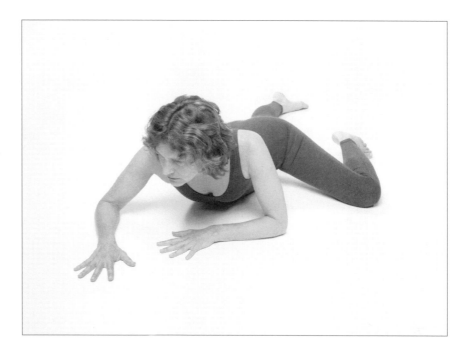

Fig. 9.4. *A homolateral crawl. The spinal side-bends are initiated by a push from the foot.* (Photograph by John Hession.)

coming up to meet you. Feel the sensations on your entire ventral surface as it contacts or is touched by the floor. Load into the belly to lift the head and chest slightly. Then rest again. Repeat the loading down and lifting up until you clearly feel that sensing the ground helps raise head and chest.

Raise the head and chest, and then the belly, off the ground, using the upper limbs for support. Notice the weight and sensation in your hands. As the belly begins to notice the support from dropping weight, the hands start to find fuller contact with the ground.

The reptile's journey out of water and onto land may feel arduous in our human body. Slow movements, dropping onto belly, chest, and cheek, then raising them again—all emphasize the energy and power required by gravity for locomotion without the ocean's support.

Lateral flexion of the spine and rib cage is still the engine for locomotion, but now the limbs transfer this force into solid ground. Begin to feel the ground through the skin of the hands and fingers and toes. Allow these sensations to feed back into the core of the body until you feel a gut connection with the ground via the hands and feet. You also touch the floor with your elbows, knees, and much of your lower leg. When a human pretends to be a lizard, more of the foreleg and forearm will touch the ground. Acknowledge that and ease your attention into toes and feet, to help stimulate the coordination of creeping on the floor.

With a sense of ground in your hands and feet, and in the belly, begin to push through one foot. Feel that push travel through the side of the body, lengthening it in a convex curve. Now the opposite leg and hip is flexed, and that opposite foot is ready to push. Again, allow the push to travel through the body. Notice that this lateral curve of the trunk also brings the upper limb of the same side forward. This is commonly referred to as homolateral movement of the spine and limbs.

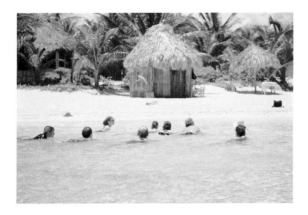 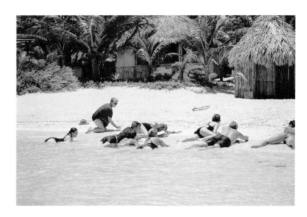

You move as the early amphibian. A soft vessel breath through slightly parted lips, flaring of the nostrils, a reptilian gaze—entering the theatre of the reptilian mind helps you embody this quality of movement. See if you can appreciate the simplicity of the gut, with an axis, slithering and pushing on land. This is the form of the amphibian and then the reptile. Dinosaurs, birds, lizards, alligators, and a vast array of other creatures followed from this innovation in form.

What was your experience moving from fish to amphibian/reptile and experimenting with lateral flexion with limbs?

Here are reports from people who have played with this transition:

One person reports: *"Each step of the way, I notice how hard it is to move! I feel clumsy and don't know what to do about it. I had started to feel some juice doing the fish movement. There was some flow. Putting my hands down, pressing into the floor felt much harder than I thought it would. I guess that's because I keep coming back to the habit of trying to 'do' the movement rather than feel the perceptions, and let the process happen. After some assistance, I realized I was letting go of my front side a little bit, and the skin of my hands could begin to notice the floor. I had a moment or two of feeling heavy and light at the same time. The mass was still in me but the effort to lift up and arch backward wasn't."*

Another person reports: *"The reptile breath (primordial breath) drew me in. I felt my nostrils flare and my gaze become cold and vacant. But inside I didn't feel cold and vacant. I felt like slithering and swinging my tail. I imagined I could reach out with my tongue and snap a bug into my body. It got to be a very simple feeling about life. Slither, eat, rest and vegetate. My brain had some down time; my thinking brain let go for a while."*

Caryn McHose recalls: *"In Mexico, at a movement retreat on a beach, the class of students spent time playing with fluid movement in the water as fish swishing, diving and swimming with their Fish Body having the feeling of no arms and legs, feeling the ease and flow of spine-generated movements. Swimming in the shallow water, beginning to play with fins turning into legs sprouting out of the side of the body and touching into the sand, students noticed the suspension of the body in the water, and their finger tips landing in the sand. They played with their fins and then with putting the limbs down, digging into the*

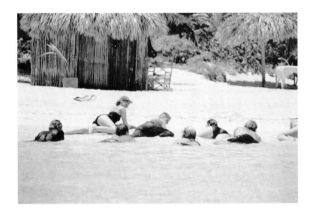

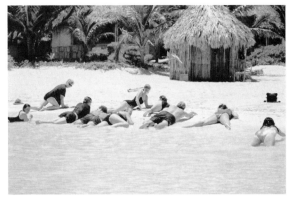

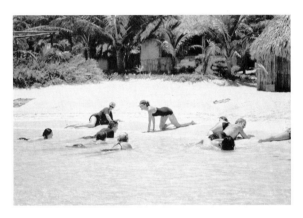

sand and pushing through the water. As students reached the water's edge, a sudden serious loading of weight into the arms and upper spine happened. At the same time they appreciated the warm sun luring them onto the sand and into the air. Some students made a U-turn and headed back into the water. Others could feel gravity loading in their bellies, in their whole body, as though for the first time, and moved fluidly up the beach."

As we move the evolutionary story, we advise slowing movements down, taking time to feel before moving, pausing during a movement. See if there is effort and see if it is possible to substitute perception for effort. When you slow down, the results are likely to be important. You may discover that your sense of weight and effort can change quite suddenly when you find support through new coordination. You may also start to enjoy the act of back-bending the trunk and suspending abdomen from limbs.

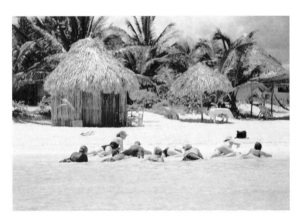

Figs. 9.5 a,b,c,d,e,f. *Movement class at beach in Tulum, Mexico.* (Photos by Carol Zickel.)

NOTES FOR TEACHERS
AND BODY THERAPISTS

Reptile and Amphibian give us the beginning of sagittal flexion and extension of the spine. We humans move with much larger sagittal flexion all the time—bending over to tie our shoe or standing up from a chair or car seat. In yoga we may do postures like the cobra, which address back-bending of the spine.

How are we back-bending, though? What is the coordination behind this movement? Are we gaining length on our front or merely contracting the back? In tonic function theory, one learns to allow the release of the antagonist before contracting the agonist. Can we release the muscles on the front of the trunk, and use the background tone of the back to bring us up? If we do, the range of motion will be greater, and the sense of effort will be less.

The contact of hands or toes on the floor is essential to release the front musculature. Learning to use hand and foot contact against an object, the floor, the wall, helps the body to lengthen. Even a small part of the fingers or hands or toes remaining out of contact will change the coordination and require effort in the back-bend.

As we work with crawling, the push of the foot against the floor is equally important. If our mind stays present to the push and the contact of the skin of the foot, the side of the body can lengthen with relative ease.

The evolutionary story follows the impulse to move into space from the first flagellate offspring of the tunicate, all the way to reptiles. Lateral flexion was first. Sagittal flexion came with the shift to being on land. Our human spine does both. Our human gait is based on a combination of both of these movements, and involves rotation as well.

Serge Gracovetsky has developed a theory about human gait and spinal mechanics he calls the spinal engine theory.[1] Gracovetsky's work has a major impact on the treatment and prevention of back pain. He describes the function of *lordosis* in the human spine and how it is regulated. The spinal engine theory explains the action of the spine—side-bending, coupled with the rotation of the sagittally curved spine—as being the force that drives walking.

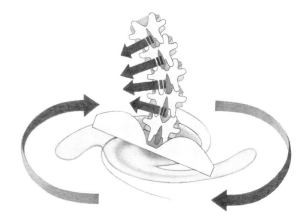

Fig. 9.6. *Side-bending of the spine produces twisting of spine and pelvis.* (Redrawn with kind permission from Serge Gracovetsky.)

Gracovetsky claims we have evolved a lordosis in our lumbar and cervical spine as a way to make upright stance possible and as a means to allow for our uniquely human gait. We can experience Gracovetsky's findings in our story of evolution. Embodying Fish Body and the subsequent experience that the fish motion drives the reptilian crawl helps open our perception to the spinal movement occurring in upright human stance.

The differentiation of spinal movement occurs best when the movement is slowed down and the dimensions of movement—that is, the side-bending, rotation, and flexion/extension of the spine—are observed and appreciated.

Differentiating spinal movement can empower the client/student in self-regulation. Fixated spinal segments are fixated because of poor coordination, stemming from trauma or poor usage patterns. When spinal movement is executed slowly, and the pre-movement is informed from perception of ground, space, and sensation of extremities, coordination has a chance to shift. This may help the spine to move more harmoniously.

Lizard movement, like that of an iguana, is different from mammal movement, like that of a cat or a dog. In the iguana, the fish body is still swishing from side to side. In the cat, it is harder to see. The spine flexes laterally and rotates. In the iguana, the limbs still look like flippers that bend around the sides of the body. In the cat, the limbs vary their extension to meet the ground, but the trunk of the cat shows a further adaptation to being on land. The changes in spinal movements give the limbs adaptability for other specialized uses. And you will never see a lizard gallop like a cat. While able to sagittally flex and extend, lizards do not use this movement to run. When they run, they look like a fish swimming.

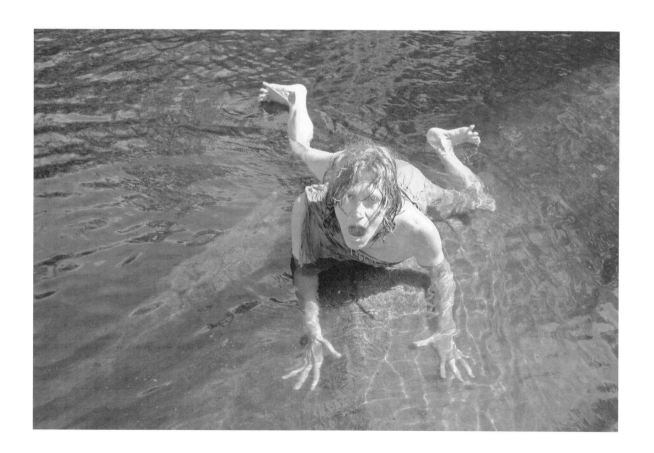

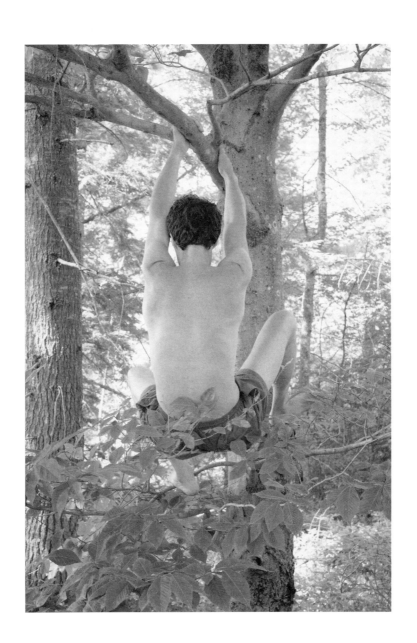

CHAPTER 10

Becoming Warm-Blooded— the Mammal

What is the difference between a lizard and a mouse? What is the difference between a crocodile and a tiger? Lizards and crocodiles are reptiles and mice and tigers are mammals. What changes occur in this evolutionary step?

In movement work, what can shifting back and forth between Reptile and Mammal teach us?

Mammals have a new approach to the function of limbs. They have warm blood, and fur. They are born fully formed and dependant on their mother for survival. Infant mammals nurse. The ribs in mammal bodies only attach to the thoracic vertebra, leaving the lumbar and cervical portions of the spine freer to move in the sagittal dimension. Mammals can express affect not only in body shape and movement, but in facial expression.

Embodying Mammal helps us rediscover movements and sensations because, as humans, we forget some of our mammalian qualities.

Orient to your sense of Mammal by reflecting on what it means to be warm-blooded. When you hear or read these words, let your mind free-associate to an image or memory, a shape, a feeling, a texture, or a sound. The image may have to do with the idea of warm-blooded or it may feel like a random association.

Take your impression and draw or journal about it. Try to move or sense into the body's response. Breathe it and, if you can, sound it. Reflect on what has come forth.

You have invoked Mammal. Read the invocations of others:

One woman says: *"When I heard you ask to think about being warm-blooded, I flashed on 'family,' a sense of the importance of my family to me. I feel my connection to my mother and father and sister and to our history. I have the image of us huddling together and sharing our warmth on a cold day in New York. The traffic noises are in the background, the sirens, honking, the buses roaring, and we are radiating warmth in our coats. I drew the picture and I'm not an artist at all, but there are four bundled shapes. To move it, I wrap my arms around myself and twist in place."*

A man also speaks about family: *"I think of my extended family and my nuclear family. Oh, we are a family. I am a son and I have a son. My father came from Greece. I am a bridge to my son who is an eager explorer of the modern American life—computers, snowboarding. I sense my arms stretching out to both of them, one on each side of me. I have long arms. I use them to play the guitar. I sing and play tunes on my guitar and that is warm-blooded."*

Another man wishes he were a reptile instead of being warm-blooded: *"Every year,*

I get depressed as the days get shorter, the nights get colder. It takes so much effort to stay warm in the winter. I wish I could let go of needing to constantly maintain my body heat. Sometimes I go to the tropics in winter. I lie down in the sun and I feel like I come alive again. What a burden to have to stay warm!

"As I go to move, I can imagine being a cold-blooded reptile, moving very slowly. No one can mess with me. I am inert and I don't have to pretend to be happy. I simply am. It's a relief to not have to relate, to maintain this Mammal business."

THE BIOLOGY OF EXPRESSION— GROWING THE MAMMAL BODY

Mammals nurse their young on the front surface of their bodies. Vaginal birth, nursing, use of forepaws and tongue to groom—all are innovations in the care of the young and the establishment of relationship. Early conditioning allows mammals to bond into lasting family and tribal groups.

Larger limbic and cortical brains, and the capacity for facial expression, make relationship more complex. A mouse can orient, can strategize its search for food and escape routes to safety. A mouse holds its bread crumb or sunflower seed in its forepaws.

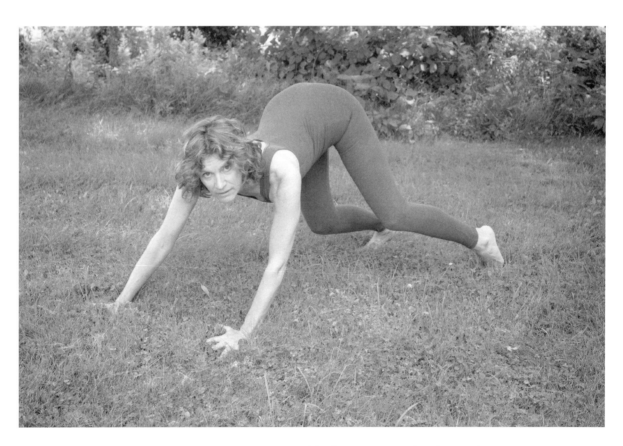

Fig. 10.2. *Exploration in orientation and facial expression as quadruped Mammal.*

The shape of Mammal changes the form of relatedness and begins to include what we recognize as expression. Primates exhibit almost human facial and verbal expression. Pets help us notice expression in other mammals. We choose to use expression as a symbol for Mammal. How do we play with the transformation from reptile to mammal?

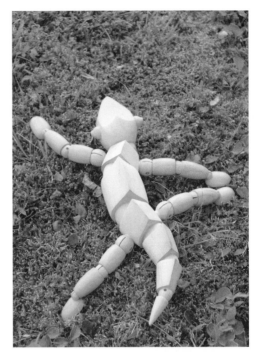

Exercise:
CHANGING THE SENSE OF LIMBS AND SPINE

Revisit your experience of Fish Body. On your belly grow the perception of a lengthening lateral line. Begin the Fish Swish and awaken lateral waves up and down the spine. Engage your limbs into the floor and raise the chest and head. Press one foot into the floor and push. The lateral line of your body, from the pushing foot to the side of the head, lengthens and bends, and at the same time travels forward on the ground. This is the homolateral crawl—the human version of the reptile's slither along the ground.

The reptile/amphibian raised its trunk from the water. How does the mammalian body make further changes in its relation to its environment? How do its limbs and girdles shift to accommodate the change?

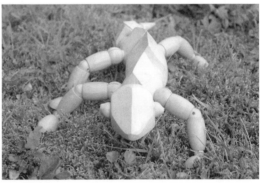

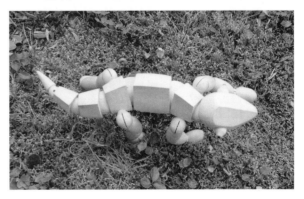

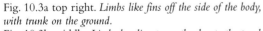

Fig. 10.3a top right. *Limbs like fins off the side of the body, with trunk on the ground.*
Fig. 10.3b middle. *Limbs bending to partly elevate the trunk.*
Fig. 10.3c lower right. *Limbs move below the body and the trunk is more elevated.*

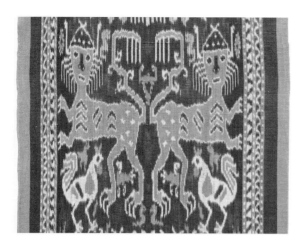

Fig. 10.4. *"Mammal Men" (detail of Indonesian textile).*

You want to establish mammalian hip and shoulder sockets, building them through your movement. On your back or side, slowly circle (circumduct) one arm at a time in its shoulder socket. Then circle one leg at a time in its hip socket. Explore the movement of the limbs in large arcs, discovering their full range of motion. Move in a clockwise and counterclockwise direction. Rest as necessary. When you pause, bring your attention to the place where your arm and thigh bones connect into their sockets. When we slowly move the range of a joint's motion it helps us feel the location and sense the joint. What happens if you alternate micro-movements with your larger ones?

Get on your hands and knees. Let your belly have its full weight so it hangs. Feel your spine's weight as well. Find and build an extension of your cone head and tail. Amplify these perceptions until it is possible to move your spine up toward the sky. Then allow it to lower. Notice that you are changing the size and shape of space between your chest/belly and the floor. As you slow this down, the limbs and front of your body take on a more mammalian movement. Imagine your arms as forelegs and your legs as hindlegs.

Tuck your toes and press them on the floor so your knees come off the floor. As you raise your hips and tail higher, feel the strength needed to power your hindlegs *(see Figures 10.5a,b)*. Feel the direction of movement that your hindlegs have and pulse your forelegs and hindlegs, bringing your trunk up and down. Rear back on your hindquarters. Notice the dimensions of movement that you are developing. Feel how the musculature of your front and back surfaces begin to engage as your spine undulates up and down, just as a cheetah does as it gallops at extraordinary speeds. Flexing and extending your trunk develops relational capacity through the front of your body *(see Fig. 10.6)*.

Return to feeling your body as a lizard. Lie down on your belly. With your hands pressed into the floor, swish side to side, letting the head and tail define the arc to right and left. Feel the lateral line of the fish that is still dominant in the lizard. Notice the closeness of your body to the ground and how your eyes scan from side to side.

Return to Mammal. Come onto your hands and knees and feel your limbs acting as props beneath you. You can contain and shift the negative space below your chest and belly. Play with ways you use your limbs and spine as the emerging mammal. You are shifting from the lateral swinging gait of the lizard to the scampering or lumbering of the mammal.

Take some time to rest and allow the sense of Mammal, the sense of affect, to arise. How do you experience this step from reptile to mammal? Can you notice the meaning of affect, or what it means to possess a warm-blooded body? Let your sensations speak to you first, allowing sensation to give rise to meaning and image.

Then, move from meaning and image to expression. Write some words or draw your image, or improvise in movement, finding what impulses the body wishes to explore.

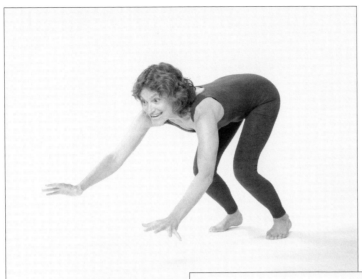

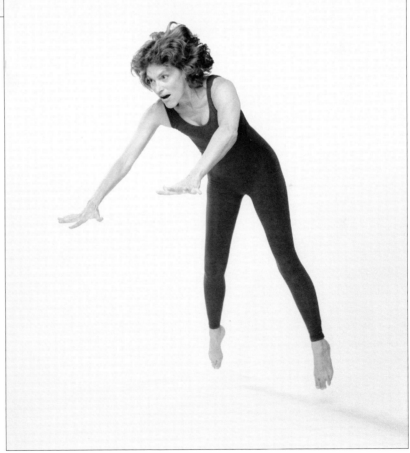

Figs. 10.5a,b. *Enjoying the pounce, feeling the power of hindlegs to propel in the direction of orientation.* (Photographs by John Hession.)

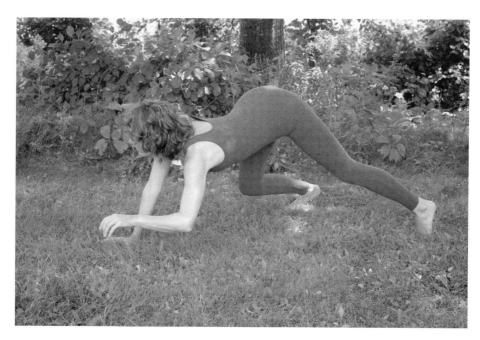

Fig. 10.6. *Flexing and extending the trunk.*

The observations of four students:

"When I did the Reptile on my belly, I felt like I was still swimming in the water, or the mud. I felt in the ground or in the swamp. Doing Mammal, I noticed I'm on top of the ground; I am up in the world. My dance is different as a mammal, because when I'm a reptile I feel like I'm just swishing side to side like a happy stupid guy who's had a little bit to drink or something. As Mammal, I've got some rhythm. I feel my shoulders like John Travolta, swaying, pushing me up and down. I feel much cooler as a mammal."

"I did the slither on the ground and then came up on my hands and knees and began to curl back, arch up like a cat. My sense of spine keeps changing. With cat back up, I get a different feeling than down in the slither mode. The feeling is a little more dangerous, a little bit more like I have an image or an identity. I have a mood. My mood feels fuller than as a reptile. I want to play with

another mammal. The lizards over there look more like food than a creature to get to know."

"The words you used to describe the mammal touched me, in a good way. The image of being nursed, of being part of a tribe or species or whatever it is that bonds the front of my body to another person, or mammal baby—that's very strong, isn't it? There's a lot of energy invested in this part of my body or to what's happening through my belly and chest, especially the chest. This probably has a big impact on our body language as mammals, as people. I started to feel how potent the space is between my chest and the ground. I was able to notice that I have strong, rich sensations in my chest as I move it above the ground, squishing the space down and then feeling the sensations as the space widens away. There is a flood of warmth and tingling when I lower down, and a sense of being pulled open as I arch up and the space gets bigger. When I stand up

and walk around, I feel how much is happening through the front of my body, approaching people, backing away. I feel like there's a lot more happening in my mammal body than I am aware of usually."

"As a lizard, my limbs are flappy things out on the side. As Mammal, I felt what you mean about haunches. There's power in the haunches! I feel like I can spring on my prey. I can pounce. And when I go back to being a lizard, I don't feel like pouncing. I feel like popping out. Pouncing is a bounce, kind of. It's having springy limbs under me."

PRIMATE—THE HU BREATH

Mammal evokes many new qualities: limb placement and use, a more sagittally articulated spine, a sense of having relationship with the front of one's body, a sense of having buttocks, of extending the tail up in the air. Mammals demonstrate different degrees of sitting up. The primate can sit and can even stand with the upper girdle free from weight bearing. She can hold her young and her young can hold onto her. The hands can perform a variety of tasks. Facial expression and vocalization allow the primate to change its countenance. The primate can communicate affect in lots of different ways.

To enter into our experience of Primate, we present the *Hu breath*. Hu breath is similar to certain yoga breaths but it has a very different intention and a somewhat different effect. The Hu breath is the invention of Emilie Conrad, the founder of Continuum.

To do the Hu breath, start by sitting comfortably on the floor, on a chair, or atop a physioball. Breathe through your mouth. On each exhale make a "ha" or "hee" or "hu" sound. Breathe continuously in and out, moderately quickly, creating a visible pumping of the belly and letting the mouth experiment with different simian expressions. Allow the rhythm of the breath to pulse the body. Play with the movement, using an imagined sense of monkey and jungle persona to inspire the shapes of the movement.

If you are on a physioball, you may start to spontaneously bounce, in counter-rhythm to the Hu breath. Experiment with letting your arms move in the air and feeling the pulse delivered in your feet. How much of your body can participate in the Hu breath?

Notice how this way of breathing and vocalizing, letting your spine and limbs move, affects your sense of body image. Compare this body image to your sense of Reptile. What novel movements follow from doing the Hu breath? What impulses arise to express these movements, to engage with another mover? What would the character of that engagement be for you?

Play in your primate body, either by yourself or with other movers. Find out the potential for action, for interaction.

If you are in a group, what unfolds? After your primate exploration, write down something that describes your experience. Then consider the following reports of other people:

"I've done the Hu breath before, in Continuum classes. I use it to warm up before I do my workout, so this isn't new to me. But I felt a new level of permission. I liked being with other movers, other monkeys. I liked the feeling of being close and playing with big dynamics, but without having to think deeply about it. I felt a sense of emotion, warmth, and playfulness without thought. When I ventured toward the cluster of other monkeys, I noticed I approached sideways, with the side of my body toward the others. I remembered the sense of the lateral line from doing the Fish Body work. I'm not sure what I was communicating, but I felt I was expressing basic feelings with my sounds, my face, and my gestures."

"The Hu breath was confusing to me—I felt somewhat stuck trying to breathe with movement of my belly. I would start to go 'hu, hu, hu' and then I ran out of breath or felt my belly get tight. What's that about?"

"My body feels tingling and sparkly, and at the same time, furry. My jaw feels rubbery and elastic. The joints of my jaw feel made out of things that are round. My lips feel thick. My hands feel full and fat. My hands want to hold other creatures close to me. Sometimes my hands and arms want to push another creature away. I like the sense of being part of a tribe."

The Hu breath can be presented in Continuum classes as a way of opening up fascia and preparing the body for changes in shape and softening of its form. Here, Hu breath is a way to feel a change of shape in our movement and meaning. We are improvising with the sense of facial mask, the gestures and cues that make up our social character, and with movements of semi-upright stance *(see Fig. 10.7)*.

The primate is a close relative to the human. Watching primate behavior, we see some of our own behaviors. By trying on the world of Primate, we see aspects of our human-ness that may not get expressed in human life. We may find gestures and body sensations that feel familiar even though we do not remember feeling them before.

Primate is a chance to find the human-ness of our being that isn't permitted by human society, but which is harmless and invigorating. The hand and face movement stimulates and innovates movement in the spine. Most important, Primate shows us how hands and facial expression add another dimension to being a mammal. Affect is the core of what we call emotion. It is arousal that supplies the energy for expression. We have played with the affect expression of Reptile and Mammal. Primate affect is more familiar to our human mind. We notice expression of affect by mice or giraffes, or even cats and dogs, and we feel we can understand it. Primate expression is closer to our own.

Primates sit up and can even stand up, although when they run they show us that they are quadrupeds by dropping onto four limbs. When they sit up we can appreciate what it means to free up the shoulders, arms, and hands from being supports.[1]

Sitting up, primates can reach out. They can push each other, grab things from each other, cover their face, and make other signals that are

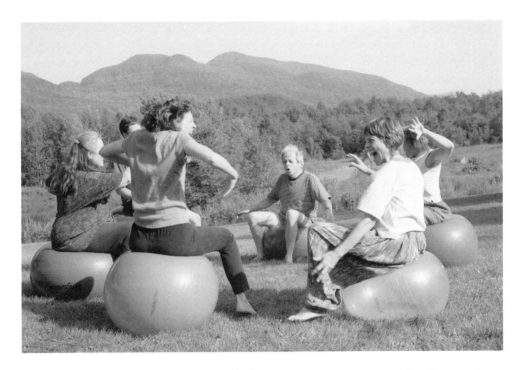

Fig. 10.7. *Exploring sound, movement, and facial expression as primates.* (Photograph by John Hession.)

not very different from our own. Primates seem to have less inhibition than we do. We address some of the differences between primates and humans in terms of healthy movement function. We want to understand the power of the human psyche that comes from linking to the tonic system.

Explore the story of your primate limbs. Feel the expressivity of your hands and the range of nuance that slight shifts of fingers and palms can take on. Touch your own face with your hands. Notice the sensitivity and refinement available to the skin of your hands and face. As a primate, your range of gesture may be enlarged because it's not part of your human story and body image.

Sense the dawning of hands, fingers, and arm movement, separate from their use as support for the trunk. You are exploring the way you can signal. You are sensing the power of gesture. Can you feel the potency of your hand out in a gesture of self-protection? Can you feel the meaning that comes from caressing and holding another person's body or head against your chest?

How does primate exploration, the Hu breath-inspired movement, affect your exploration of hand gesture? Can you switch back to human mind for a moment? Can you feel the modern human hands that go to punch in a telephone number, or that operate a car? What happened for you to make that switch? What are the qualities that give you the familiar sense of examining hand, fingers, arm, and gesture, as a modern human? If you switch back to the Primate sense, how did you do that? What helped you make that change?

Rotate the attention between the two polarities; feel your imagined primate hand. Then feel your human hand. The transition informs meaning. Meaning informs movement. Culture informs meaning. Our sense of culture comes from observing the movements of our tribe.

What happens if you include your legs and feet as equally expressive? Let the soles of your feet and the palms of your hands touch each other. Can the feet and hands exchange roles as toucher and receiver? How do your feet meet the world with expression and gesture?

The world of Primate lets us explore movement forms and anatomical details uncoupled from our human meanings. We can observe how our manners and gestures are formed by our culture. We sense our gestures as cultural when we notice that they are automatic but not inherent. When we feel our ability to do primate gesture, freely and easily, we realize that as humans we have a huge potential vocabulary and we only use a tiny part of it. We are habituated to our territory and social group. This is the fourth structure of tonic function theory. Meaning structure shapes our movement potential.

NOTES FOR TEACHERS AND BODY THERAPISTS

Investigations of Primate, the Hu breath, and warm-bloodedness allow people to explore the roots of musculoskeletal issues. Our aches and pains and chronic tension syndromes in many parts of the body are rooted in our human dilemma. How do I keep civilization, which is necessary and good, from arresting my creativity and freedom of expression?

Of course, there is no answer. It is a dialectic between form and flow. We need language and rules and social structure to organize our means of survival. We need flow or we start to stifle—psychologically, physically, physiologically, and spiritually.

Flow without form might be like a drunken dancer. Form without flow is controlled but stiff. Flow without form is an attempt to avoid a basic human quality—the ability to drive on the same side of the road as an example. Without it we die. Form without flow is an attempt to avoid impulses and creativity. If we are in charge of a school or company and create too many rules and enforce them, our employees will hate their jobs.

Alternating between human and primate gesture, we notice our tendencies about form and flow. When students observe primate hand and then human hand, what happens? Do they see flow in the human hand? Do they resist letting go of familiar movements?

This work is about finding mutability of forms, not learning to have a new, better form. We gain flexibility in our qualities of movement, our forms, by accidents of new perception. When we discover a brand new movement, the form-versus-flow question flies out the window. We are alive. We move with flow and form and neither is a problem.

We work with observation. That is the beginning of change. If the exploration is supplied with meaning, imagination, breath, and attention to sensation, we will have accidents of perception that allow the body to do something new.

In our consideration of Mammal, in this case the primate, we touch parts of the body where many people have issues. Shoulder and neck complaints, TMJ, carpal tunnel syndrome, tension headaches, and eye strain are a few of the maladies found in the face, neck, shoulder, and arms.

In order to improve someone's function, a holistic practitioner needs to assist the client/student in uncoupling body image from the experience of movement. Hu breath is hard for some people to imagine doing at first. Many have to titrate such an experience, taking tiny steps toward this adventure. To the degree that someone is comfortable, the contrast of human hand and face with primate hand and face is a provocative and dynamic approach. Whenever we give birth to a new movement from orientation and sense impression we loosen the hold of body image over our movement.

SHIFTING PERCEPTIONS

Doing Hu breath, perhaps you found yourself moving your jaw, lips, and eyes in ways that felt different. You may also have found unusual sensations afterwards. If you notice sensations, follow them. They may shift. You might notice other parts of the body, or a different aspect of the room around you. You are using breath, sound, movement, meaning, and imagination to shift your perception.

You shift your perception in the direction of sensations in the face. Our bodies have a huge proportion of sensory receptors in the hands, feet, and face. Many fewer sensory receptors inhabit the back or the calf. We have sensory receptors in areas of nuanced movement. In fact, improvement of fine motor skill of any body region requires improvement in the flow of sensory information in that part of the body.

Improved attention to sensation helps us move in finer ways. Why is this so?

Body image is the conscious and unconscious body map that lives inside us. It is a powerful force on how we move. If my parent tells me something about my body over and over—something like "you have a very large butt"—I start to hold a picture or feeling of a large bottom. Coupled with that image will be an opinion about that image. Some part of my consciousness will either be devoted to "I should try to minimize or hide my butt" or perhaps "I have a wonderful large butt, I will show it off." In either case, I don't have to think those words consciously for them to influence posture and movement.

My body image guides my coordination and my quality of movement. There are more subtle examples. Dancers, who are taught to think about having a pelvis, will move as though the pelvis and adjacent structures are a single unit. They may move competently, with proper form, but there will be a blocked flow between the leg and spine. If a dancer is taught to think about the legs being connected to the spine at the level of the twelfth thoracic vertebra, the movement will look different. This is a principle of body image instruction that is common in the practice of Structural Integration. Change the body image and you change the movement. However, you can directly change some body image issues and not others. Sometimes the body image is tenacious. What then?

Consider again Godard's four components to body structure.[2] The first is physical structure—the bones, ligament, and fascia. The second component is perceptual. Perceptive structure is the tendency to keep using sensory channels in familiar ways. Perceptive structure keeps us using our sensory and attentional system in similar grooves. The third component is coordination. Coordinative structures are the acquired subroutines that make complex recruitment and timing decisions when we perform any action. If we reach for and lift a glass of water to our lips, our body decides automatically how to get this job done. The fourth component is meaning structure. Our culture, our environment, our family, and individual experience, all take part in codifying our movements.

All four structures are at work in determining the way we move in any given circumstance.

The "lock" on the structure of our movement is not meant to be unlocked casually. If it could be unlocked easily, we would be vulnerable to failure when our lives depend on movement to function automatically, for our survival.

To unlock the structure of our body movement and posture, we explore shifts of perception, including body image and meaning. We also hope for happy accidents of coordination. If you can communicate with the latter three structures, physical structure is the easiest to change.

Why does attention to sensation help us shift our places of habitual movement? Body image is very powerful. To become aware of the deeply ingrained and taboo parts of our body image we need to give the coordinative part of our brain abundant sensory information. It is sensory perception that helps unlock the body image.

Hands and face and front of the body are capable of complex and expressive relational dynamics. The hands and face are richly endowed with sense receptors. Using the Hu breath and Primate exploration gives an opportunity to communicate by invoking expressive gesture involving hands, face, and front of the body.

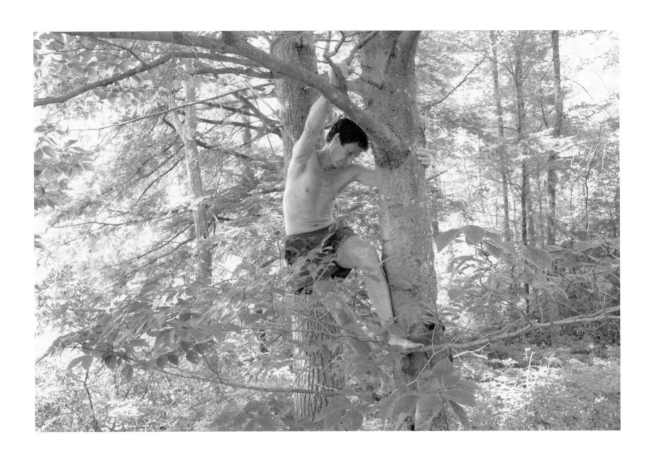

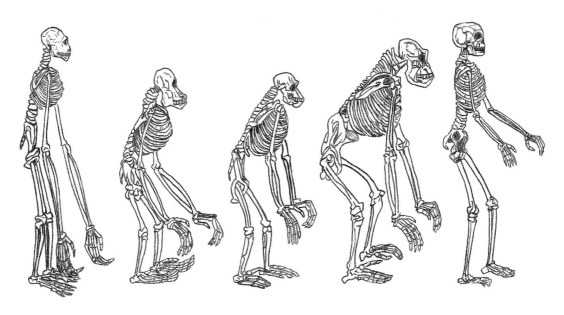

Fig. 11.1. *Comparison of human and primate skeletal structures. Left to right: gibbon, orangutan, chimpanzee, gorilla, man.* (Redrawn from Waterhouse Hawkins drawing of skeletons in Museum of the Royal College of Surgeons, circa 1850.)

CHAPTER 11

The Human—
Walking Upright, Achieving Lordosis

If you can read this page you are probably human. Human beings organize through language and sets of rules based on the ability to count and make symbolic distinctions. Humans use the past to make movement predictions about the future.[1] Humans live in a thought-created reality, at least much of the time. Symbolic reality seems to be a particular tendency of humans.

Humans can become aware that thinking is occurring. Contemplative traditions explore the possibility of awareness without the intervening movie screen of thought. Movement study can help us explore this kind of awareness. Movement study can lead to happy accidents of what Toni Packer describes as "seeing without knowing."[2]

It is helpful to become aware that symbolic meaning has a grip on our movement. With awareness, we have some chance of shifting movement patterns.

For centuries, and perhaps millennia, human beings have asked themselves, "Is it possible to be free of the world that my mind has made up?" You are encouraged to wonder. Notice how meanings operate with regard to movement. To what degree can we notice the power and the shapes of our meaning structures? Meaning shape is always guiding movement shape.

We ask the question, "What makes human movement interesting and different from the other creatures we have looked at?" What about human movement led to this large brain and all the details of human life this brain made possible?

There are numerous body qualities that are different from primates and from other mammals. If you see a human being wearing a gorilla costume running for his life, you would know he is, in fact, a human in a gorilla suit and not a bona fide gorilla.

If you watch a cat, dog, squirrel, horse, or rabbit walk, what do you see their spine do? Having moved like a fish, a lizard, and a mammal, can you see what the spine of the mammal is doing when it walks? Primarily you will see lateral flexion (like a fish). You will also see the spine lifting up and down. Finally, you will see some twisting occur. The hips and shoulders travel up and down and the spine twists to help this, then untwists releasing energy back. Fish motion (lateral flexion) and torsion (twisting) go together in mammalian spines.

When you watch a cat, dog, or rabbit run, what do you see? What does their spine do? Or watch a horse, a cheetah, or a whale. The spine elongates and contracts in a forward and backward manner *(see Figs. 11.2a,b)*. This is called *homologous spinal*

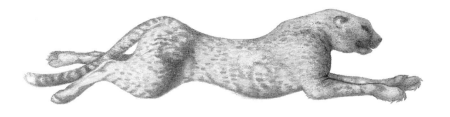

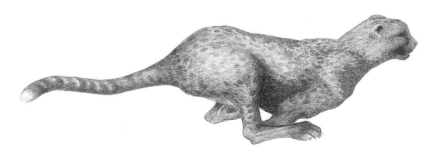

Figs. 11.2a,b. *Drawings of cheetah running, with locomotion showing sagittal flexion of the spine.* (Drawings by Galen Beach).

movement. The two sides of the spine are doing the same motion. We also call this spinal motion *sagittal flexion* (and extension). A quadruped uses this strategy to go the fastest. The quadruped's spinal power is greatest when used as one big spring.

Humans run on two legs. They run based on the spinal motions of the fish. When running, the human spine bends side to side and, as with all mammals, the spine also bends forward and backward. The human spine twists around its longitudinal axis. The pelvis and lower spine rotate to one side and the upper spine and shoulders rotate in the opposite direction. In walking and running the human spine moves in three ways—side to side, forward and backward, and rotation and counter-rotation.

Other mammal spines also rotate. Human spines, however, rotate and counter-rotate with an upper girdle that doesn't bear weight and with a spine oriented vertically. We can call this manner of walking *contralateral gait*.

It is hard to observe spine movement separate from limb movement. Begin this exploration by letting your body differentiate spine from limb movement by spending time on all fours. See if you can feel the combination of lateral flexion and twisting in your spine.

LORDOSIS

Why do humans do something different than quadrupeds when they run? Humans can stand truly upright and walk and run that way because of the shape of their spine. Looking at our spines from the side, you notice several curves *(see Fig. 11.3).* You see two places of lordosis and three places of kyphosis. It is *lordosis*, in particular, that we wish to focus on.

Think about the word *lordosis.* What does this idea mean to you? What does it evoke? Write down, or draw the meaning that comes to you. Then experiment with moving that meaning. This gives you a baseline. If you know your baseline of meaning, new ideas can be considered.

What is your baseline for thinking about lordosis? Consider the stories of some other students:

"A therapist told me I have a lordosis. He told me that that's why I get back pain. I looked in the mirror and looked at photographs and he was right. My back bends in and pushes my belly forward. I've worked at pushing it back, doing sit-ups and standing with my back against the wall, pressing the hollow part against the wall. I'm not really sure that it's helped. I'm annoyed in my body when I think about lordosis. It's a sensation of restlessness, tightness in my legs. I drew a picture of a stick person and the curve is way forward in the low back. There are red jagged lines in the legs and around the head and neck and spine and belly. I am wondering now if my back is just pushed too far forward and it's stuck that way."

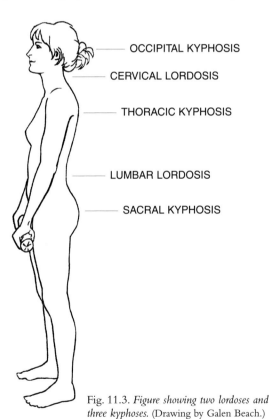

OCCIPITAL KYPHOSIS

CERVICAL LORDOSIS

THORACIC KYPHOSIS

LUMBAR LORDOSIS

SACRAL KYPHOSIS

Fig. 11.3. *Figure showing two lordoses and three kyphoses.* (Drawing by Galen Beach.)

Another report: *"There was a time when I read Ida Rolf's book, and got a series of sessions. I got the impression that the point of Structural Integration was to make the lordosis smaller. The book said you need to 'horizontalize' your pelvis. I got some work from other practitioners and one of them said I need to have more lordosis in my back, that I was too flat. So, I started to work at letting my belly go and being okay with a curve. I watched a slide show that a yoga teacher showed of bodies around the world. The indigenous people from Africa and Australia had deep curves—deep lordosis in their low backs. Now, the rage is to do Pilates and get your curve to go back. I'm starting to realize that I'm not going to find an answer as to whether to have a lordosis or not. I think the curves have to fit each person and what he or she is doing, and they can't be stuck in one position or another. There has to be flexibility and at the same time there has to be stability. It's tricky.*

"I moved my lordosis up and down. As I moved I realized how 'in your head' you can get about these ideas. It feels clear that when I move my spine forward and backward, slowly, the movement gets easier and the pieces of the spine articulate better. It feels like my answer for now is to get even and separated movement."

A horse rider trained to find her "seat" reports: *"Lordosis is the thing that happens when you let your back move forward too much. I have worked to control that, to feel the sense of dropping my sit bones down through the horse. I drew a picture of a body on a horse with the line from the ear to the sit bone down through the body of the horse to the ground. I can feel that sense in my body as I look at the picture."*

Another student reports: *"Lordosis sounds like a disease. I started to play with the word and it led to 'lardosis,' someone with a lot of lard in their belly. I walked around with a feeling of lard making my belly stick out, and feeling heavy."*

A singer tells us that she is "swaybacked" and because of that she can't get enough breath for her singing. She recognized that lordosis was related to the being sway-backed. She is wondering how to fix her swayed back.

If you feel confused about the concept of lordosis, you are not alone. There is an ongoing debate about lordosis in the bodywork and orthopedic world. The origin of the word appears to be from Old English, meaning "to deceive," and from Greek, meaning "bending forward." Webster's defines it as "abnormal curvature of the spine forward." This raises the question, what is normal and abnormal curvature?

Lordosis can be a confusing idea, but without this shape we wouldn't be human and we couldn't walk or run the way we do. Lordosis is central to our movement.

A more lengthy discussion of lordosis appears at the end of this chapter. In general terms, however, we need to understand some basic facts about spine shape and movement to appreciate the dilemma of human gait and posture.

trunk. This is the origin of the primary curves of the back, the curves of the thoracic spine (the part of the spine with ribs) and the head and sacrum. Our spine starts out with this shape.

How do humans end up with concave curves in the neck and low back? The answer is that we develop these secondary curves from impulses of relationship—relationship to all the elements of the space around us. We build our shape as we reach out to our world. In our reaching out to touch, to grasp, to better orient, we grow our secondary curves.

What is the developmental movement that shapes the human spine? There are different kinds of changes that occur: perceptual steps, anatomical growth, learning to make contact and push with limbs. Child development specialists have studied this process and we won't attempt to summarize their work. Here, we only consider some of the movements that shape our spines.

THE HUMAN SPINE

Look at the illustration of a human skeleton next to various primates at the beginning of this chapter. Look at the shape of the spine, the way the body curves in the backbone. Notice the shift that occurred in the lumbar curve as we see modern human next to his ancestors.

Human beings have a definite concave curve in the low back and the neck. These concave curves are each a lordosis of the spine. In the upper back, the head, and the sacrum, the curves are convex. Look at the picture of the human embryo *(see Fig. 11.4)*. In the womb, we develop as a creature with one long curve of the head and

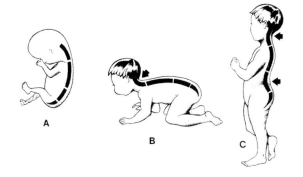

Fig. 11.4. *Early stages of spinal development. A: primary curve of fetus. B: secondary curve developing in the neck. C: secondary curve in low back and neck. (Redrawn with kind permission from Serge Gracovetsky.)*

REACHING

What forms the shape of our spine? Start by asking yourself the question, "What does reaching out mean?" Either write or move your association with reaching. Do you have an association that includes enticement? Can you remember or imagine an incident where you were enticed to reach out?

After you have some felt sense of reaching out, and have noticed at least one manner in which you relate to this, consider some others:

"I am asleep. A giant lump lands on my body and then stays there on four paws pressing into my chest. I think, 'oh, the cat is saying it's time to get up and feed me.' I lie still. The cat is watching me, I can tell. I lie still. Now, through my half-closed lids, I see the cat extend a paw very slowly toward my face. The pads of the paw touch my cheek. The cat withdraws its paw. I lie still. The cat's paw extends out again, slowly moving toward my cheek. The pads touch and then I feel the points of his claws emerge from the paw and make tiny dents in my face. I guess I'm getting up now."

"I used to get up each morning, in a different part of my life, and milk the cow and shovel out the barn. As I milked and shoveled, I slowly woke up. I wheeled the manure and straw to the little field and used a fork to throw the manure out on the field. When the stuff left the fork and flew through the air, I felt a feeling like something was flying out of my belly, into the winter air. I did a gesture of this and it's still easy to feel it."

"I see someone hurting and I feel my body get lighter. I feel my chest move forward. I see an image of my hands reaching out to comfort. I see something beautiful on the beach and I feel my hand being drawn toward it, like a magnet, my hand, my eyes, my mouth even if it isn't something to eat. I do the movement and I feel myself

drawn by an imagined object of interest, and I let my chest move and fall back and my fingers stretch out and then relax. My neck undulates with each rising and reaching and falling back."

"A one-year-old girl sits in her high chair. She sees the cup and reaches forward to grab it and pulls it toward her and it falls over. She looks up at her mother with big eyes. Seeing the cup leads to reaching and grabbing. Feeling the cup fall, she reaches with her eyes toward her mother. She is curious and eager to touch the world. Her eyes appear to reach out and ask a silent question."

Consider the role of reaching out in the development of body shape. Does your experience relate to the meaning and movement of development we describe?

THE HUMAN INFANT'S DILEMMA

Babies start to explore as soon as they are held. They are curious. They need to be curious, as most mammals do, to survive. They need to find food and they need to sort out what works to be safe, warm, and cared for. They are curious because that is the nature of being. They are responsive to novelty, and at the beginning everything is new.

Babies differ in their orientation to other. Some are more aggressive at finding the breast, or a toy or other object, using their hands, using their voice. Some babies are quieter and more passive, and there are combinations of action and receptivity.

The movement of reaching with the mouth and hands begins right away. Reaching with the mouth and hand brings the spine and shoulder into a shape. That shape, if repeated, will start to form the shape of the baby's body.

Fast-forward now to the beginnings of loco-motion: babies begin by pushing with their feet.

At this point, the baby is lying with its belly on the floor. The foot on one side finds some traction and pushes the body forward on one side. This action reveals fish-like movement of the spine. The trunk bends to one side as the body is propelled forward.

Babies start to look up while lying on their belly. Try doing that. What happens to the shape of your neck? Our perception guides our movement. Movement leads to shape. Over time the shape of our movement results in structure.

At some point, a baby gains altitude, not by standing but by sitting up. She or he also becomes a quadruped by crawling (creeping) on all fours, the hands and knees. This crawl is different than that of the reptile.

Exercise:
CRAWLING (CREEPING) AND REACHING

Begin to move on your hands and knees. (You may want knee protection.) If you are part of a group, divide the group in half, so half can watch, and then switch after a bit. See if you can see the motion of the trunk. Does the trunk move as one unit? Does the trunk have segments that move in different ways? Can you see mammal movement (sagittal flexion) or fish movement (lateral flexion)?

This is your baseline. It might be helpful to draw or note what you saw.

Take your quadruped position again. Now reach out with your gaze. Look in the near distance at something interesting. Reach for it with your hand. We need to arouse genuine interest in reaching for our body to respond. Reach out slowly enough to notice what happens to the shape of your spine.

Did your spine change shape? Did it curve upward or downward, or to one side? Typically a

reach will draw the spine into an extended shape. Thus, as you reach out with your hand, you may feel your neck get a deeper curve, or you may find that your low back gets a deeper curve; you may find that your chest moves farther from your belly.

Reaching out with your hand has a similar effect to reaching out with your eyes, ears, or nose. Reaching out with the senses is part of our desire to know the world around us. Reaching out is also an effort to touch or grasp the world. As humans, our arms, head, and chest have great freedom to reach. As we reach, our bodies gain in their capacity to extend.

When we reach out with our desire or our eyes and hand, we build the curve, or lordosis, in our low back and neck. There is variety in the amount of curve people have in their low backs and necks. Some of this variation is probably genetic. Some is acquired by modeling, by contexts that support or inhibit reaching out or back-bending of the trunk.

We build our human-shaped spine through our early life. Reaching out, in human fashion, builds our particularly human-shaped spine.

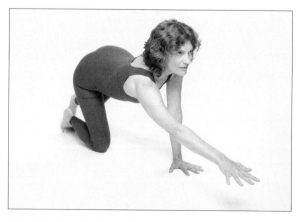

Fig. 11.5. *Crawling (creeping) on all fours, initiated with reaching.* (Photograph by John Hession.)

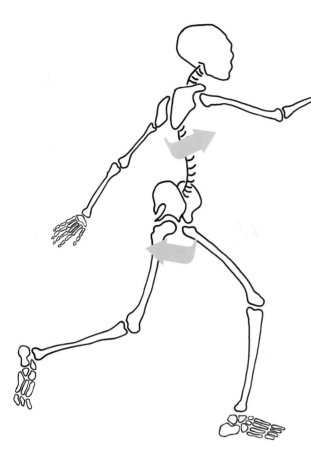

Fig. 11.6. *Schematic of human gait.*
(Drawing by Susan Kress Hamilton.)

HUMAN SHAPE AND HUMAN WALK

Gracovetsky,[3] in his spinal engine theory, asserts that humans have made a particular adaptation for upright locomotion and the development of lordosis in our spine has enabled this adaptation.

Our lordotic spine converts fish body motion (lateral flexion) into rotation and counter-rotation in the lower and upper spine and girdles. We walk in something known as contralateral gait *(see Fig. 11.6).*

The spine's shape, the tendency to move from side to side, and to rotate and counter-rotate, combine to be one of the key evolutionary steps that denote human being. The lordotic curves are the foundation to the upright stance, the upright locomotion. Why then does lordosis get such a bad reputation?

Once upon a time lordosis was an admired trait. If we look not just at aboriginal cultures, but also at paintings of people through the ages, lordotic curves are a part of the accepted, even admired, human form.

Modern attitudes toward the shape of the spine seem to have shifted during the twentieth century. The influence of such things as physical education and dance training, the reduction of walking, the search for a cure for back pain have led to the belief that excess lordosis is the problem.

BACK PAIN

During an episode of back pain, it is instinctive to contract the belly wall, the pelvic floor, and the buttock muscles to splint against painful movement. Many fitness classes and some therapists recommend this as a strategy to prevent back injury. People easily get the impression that lumbar lordosis is the enemy of back health.

Ida Rolf proposed a holistic solution to back pain, but unfortunately some of her ideas helped foster the notion that the lumbar spine should be somewhat flattened. The illustrations in her book *Rolfing: Reestablishing the Natural Alignment and Structural Integration of the Human Body for Vitality and Well-Being* imply that a horizontal pelvis (one that reduces lordosis) is an important goal.

Core stabilization exercise classes can give students the impression that a healthy spine is one that is pushed back in the lumbar area.

THE MIND OF IDEALS

There is a difference between posture that is based on an abstract ideal and posture that is responsive to circumstance, that arises out of context.

Lordosis of the spine is naturally regulated by the stabilizer muscles of the trunk—that is, until certain forms of thought get involved. When we think about abdominal muscles and about stabilizing our lordosis, we control our posture consciously and create fixation. Even thinking about our abdomen is likely to activate the superficial belly wall. These muscles pull the chest down and, when habitually contracted, lead to weakening of the deeper system that supports us in dynamic movement. Coupled with belly wall tightening is buttock tightening and pelvic floor tightening.

Lordosis does need regulation. Muscles that increase lordosis need to be balanced by muscles that decrease lordosis.

The circumferential muscles of the abdomen work like a belt around the lower trunk. They are called the transversus abdominus. The deep muscles of the central spine, the multifidus group, function to erect the spine. Together these two groups of muscles work to control lordosis. This occurs in contralateral gait as well as when the trunk is challenged to stabilize itself.

Well-intentioned therapists or fitness instructors teach students to activate their core-stabilizing muscles with words such as "press your spine back" or, in the dance world, "squeeze your buttock muscles." There are many variations to these often counterproductive instructions.

The result is a population that feels a lordotic spine is a weak spine, that lordosis is something to inhibit. We considered this issue in Chapter 6 on the gut body when we played with having a belly.

How can we rehabilitate postural integrity of the spine? Moving from a sense of space and weight by activating sense impression in the extremities serves us well in spinal stabilization.

Have you ever climbed a tree or a jungle gym? Or painted something almost out of reach while standing on a ladder? In such circumstances your body is trying to reach something while stabilizing with the other three limbs. If you have climbed, ask yourself if you would contract your abdomen at the same time. Does it make any sense? Imagine contracting your belly, buttocks, or your pelvic floor while standing on a ladder with a bucket of paint in one hand and the brush reaching out in the other. Does it feel like an intelligent move?

Fortunately, our bodies are much smarter than our thinking mind. Otherwise, our species wouldn't have made it this far. When you climb, your hands and feet and sense of being in mid-air

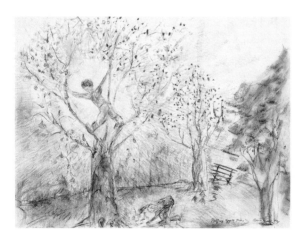

Fig. 11.7. *"Rolfing Apple Trees."* (Pastel/watercolor by Bonnie Bell.)

are wired to activate the appropriate trunk-stabilizing muscles. This stabilization prevents collapse while ensuring flexibility so that you can move around like a monkey.

This capacity to move and be stabilized is often not functioning well in human beings. Especially for those who have suffered back pain episodes, there is an interruption in this mechanism. Then, lordosis is not properly regulated. When stability has been interrupted, there will be weakness in recruitment of stabilizer muscles. Then we must re-teach the body to regulate itself, to let go of unhelpful habits of squeezing and tightening so we can rekindle the activity that efficiently and gracefully supports the trunk.

Exercise:
FLIGHT OF THE EAGLE

Flight of the Eagle is an exercise that will help you find core stability. You will learn to stabilize by using perception and orientation to weight and space. You need a bench or a low table to put your hands on.

Place your hands on the bench, shoulder-width apart. Place your feet on the floor, shoulder-width apart. Your feet are in line with your buttocks. Your legs are straight. Your arms are straight and your hands are about a foot beyond your head. The position is illustrated below. Arrows illustrate "vectors of perception"—perceptions of direction into space, and places of sensory impression in the hands and feet *(see Fig. 11.8)*.

Start your movement by noticing the ground. Sense where your body can load and feel weight. Notice your orientation to space, the aspects of yourself that can sense surrounding space. Each time you begin, this pre-movement enlivens the sensory channels that help to orchestrate effective movement.

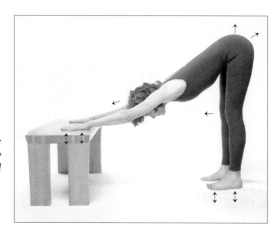

Fig. 11.8. *Flight of the Eagle, starting position. The arrows indicate "vectors of perception" into space. Double-headed arrows show simultaneous sense impressions received by hands and feet, and pressing of hands and feet on bench or floor.*
(All photographs of this exercise by John Hession.)

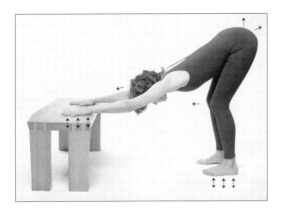

Fig. 11.9. *Flight of the Eagle.*

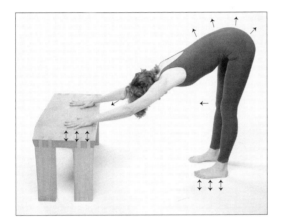

Fig. 11.10. *Flight of the Eagle.*

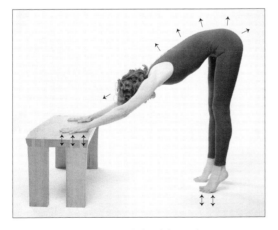

Fig. 11.11. *Flight of the Eagle.*

To begin Flight of the Eagle, find and receive sense impression in your feet and hands. Allow the texture, mass, and temperature of what you are touching to be received through your hands and feet. By letting in sense impression, your body starts to notice its context more deeply. The flow of noticed sensation orients the body to flow in movement.

Notice how your hands and feet press in the direction of the ground. Also notice the direction of your sit bones lifting toward the sky. Notice your knees sensing the space in front of them. Amplify the direction of your knees forward into space until they move that way, but still maintain the directions of the feet, hands, and sit bones *(see Fig. 11.9)*. Amplify your sense of sit bones reaching to sky and feet pressing into the ground until your knees extend. Knees continue to feel their forward direction. No senses of direction need be lost as you amplify others.

Refresh your sense of hands and feet as they contact the floor and bench and your sit bones as they lift into space. How much of your skin body can notice the potency of the surrounding space? Allow your eyes to be soft and receive peripherally. Shift your ground contact slightly, from the heel into forefoot, and allow a little more press of the hands into the bench *(see Fig. 11.10)*. The sit bones still reach for sky. The head is sensing omni-directionally, alive to space. The body will lift off and be supported in the toes and the hands *(see Figs. 11.11 and 11.12).*

Continue to lift off and come forward until your weight is mostly on your hands. Perhaps you feel your trunk lifted as if from some other force, not your own. Refresh your hands' sense of bench and then push into the bench, making maximum skin contact with your fingers and palms. Pressing the hands should press the spine back, releasing the spinal segments to emerge behind you. Pressing your hands will also allow you to amplify the toe pressure into the floor. Pressing hands and feet together allows the spine to feel like a bent spring as it presses out on its convex surface *(see Fig. 11.13).*

Feel your spine as a bent spring. Feel hands and feet and their contact to bench and floor. Feel a broad sense of space. As you press a little more with your hands, you will deliver weight to your feet and land on the whole length and breadth of your feet *(see Fig. 11.14).*

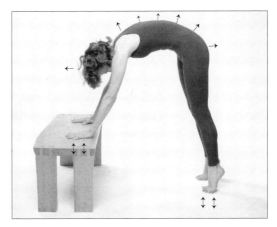

Fig. 11.12. *Flight of the Eagle.*

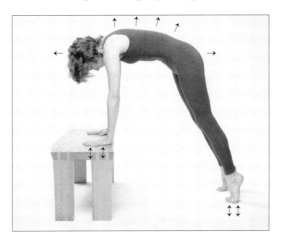

Fig. 11.13. *Flight of the Eagle.*

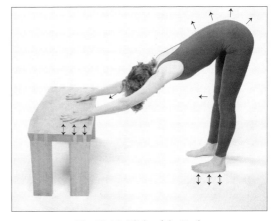

Fig. 11.14. *Flight of the Eagle.*

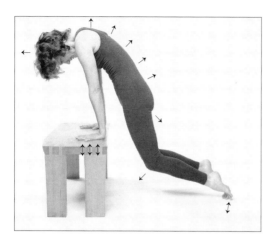

Fig. 11.15. *Flight of the Eagle.*

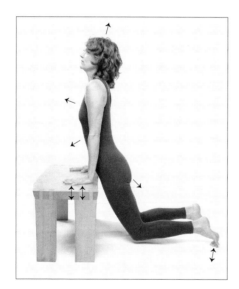

Fig. 11.16. *Flight of the Eagle.*

Reestablish skin contact with hands and feet and the perception of knee and sit bone directions into space. Raise your weight onto your toes by amplifying your sit bone direction toward the sky. When you have lifted up and forward onto your hands, let your knees drop down toward but not touching the floor *(see Fig. 11.15).*

You are supported by hands and toes but your body is allowed to hang in a long open curve *(see Fig. 11.16).* Now activate sense impression in your hands again. Refresh sense impression and notice the power of doing so.

Press the bench strongly with the skin of your hand, so the skin is active. Emphasize your finger tips and then sequence your pressure along your fingers toward your palms. Link the sense of fingers to the cervical vertebra as you begin the sequence through the spine *(see Fig. 11.17).* Press your toes into the floor and allow your spine to articulate its vertebral segments starting with the atlas and sequencing each spinal segment from top to bottom *(see Fig. 11.18).* Each segment of the spine notices its sense of sky, and lifts toward the sky, as the hands and feet supply the ground *(see Fig. 11.19).* Allow the hands to deliver the differentiated spine back down into the heels.

As an experiment, try this exercise with your belly wall intentionally contracted. Then do it with only hands and feet making contact with ground, sit bones and knees finding a sense of direction, and the whole body feeling alive to space. Alternate between the two until you feel clear about the contrast. When you feel this contrast clearly, you will have an insight into the natural source of core stabilization.

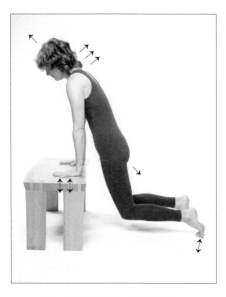

Fig. 11.17. *Flight of the Eagle.*

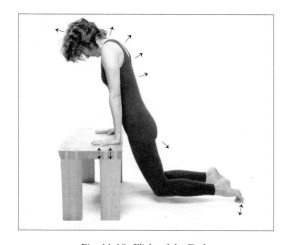

Fig. 11.18. *Flight of the Eagle.*

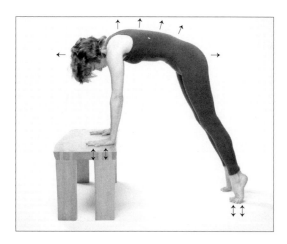

Fig. 11.19. *Flight of the Eagle.*

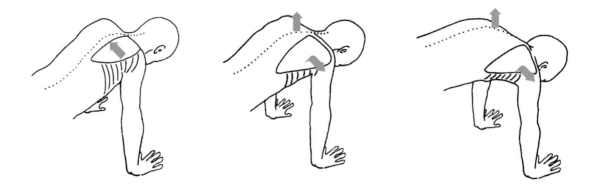

Fig. 11.20. *The serratus anterior muscle stabilizes the shoulder blade and articulates the trunk from the shoulder. This is the muscle uniquely able to stabilize the shoulder girdle.* (Drawing by Susan Kress Hamilton.)

FLIGHT OF THE EAGLE AND LORDOSIS

The spine can flex and extend, bending forward and backward in a way that allows it to be flexible and strong at the same time. Movement in the Flight of the Eagle changes our spine from a lordotic shape to a more kyphotic shape without contraction of the belly in the conventional sense. The belly may lift and hollow out, the curve of the back may change from concave to convex—yet we are not thinking about doing something with the belly wall. The deep layer of the belly wall—the transversus abdominus—is triggered to contract because the body calls for stability from the hands and feet. Hands and feet are saying, in effect, "Give me support so I can press against the floor and the bench to power the body in space."

Lordosis gets regulated naturally. However, sometimes the body's responses for stabilizing itself need rehabilitation. The Flight of the Eagle can revive natural regulation.

Flight of the Eagle teaches us that the trunk is also stabilized by the shoulder-stabilizing muscle known as serratus anterior. The serratus anterior muscle *(illustrated above)* is part of the body's stabilizing system. The shoulder blade travels forward on the rib cage through the action of the serratus shortening and the rhomboids lengthening. In Flight of the Eagle, the serratus is essential for pressing the spine into the air and catching it again as it drops toward the Earth.

Serratus action is a specific part of upper body stabilization. It is triggered by sensory impression in the hands coupled with differentiated orientation to weight and space. When we trigger the serratus, we help make it easier to trigger the transversus and multifidus as well. By turning on intrinsic shoulder and upper trunk stabilization, it is easier to turn on other parts of the stabilizing system.

A student with back pain had the following comments after practicing Flight of the Eagle for several weeks:

"A small amount of the Eagle means I can bend over at the waist without difficulty. It's nice to get length in my hamstrings without focusing on them. Sometimes you don't know where to put your shoulders, where to put your body. This feels like a 'guiding' for your spine so that you feel it's attached to your legs. You feel young again. Everything is in its place, rather than the old man thing. [He mimics the posture of someone bent over because of back pain or old age.] *When the spine goes forward and backward, it feels like a 'cleaning out' of the spine. It's like a bellows with the front of the spine fattening up and then blowing out and then the back of the spine fattening up and blowing out. Everything gets cleaned out."*

Stabilizing activity is a system dynamic. We either turn on the system or we don't. Turning on the system is a natural consequence of engagement with our environment, with ground and sky, with handles, tools, and tree branches, with animals, people, plants, and water. Sensory engagement and orientation to the world around us stimulates the body's stabilizing system.

Fig. 11.21. *Receiving sense impression in the hands and feet liberates movement from the confines of body image. Working this way, there may be moments in which, oriented deeply through our hands and feet to the world around us, we find the sense of body relatively empty, relatively free of the burden of self-concern.* (Photograph by Jay O'Rear.)

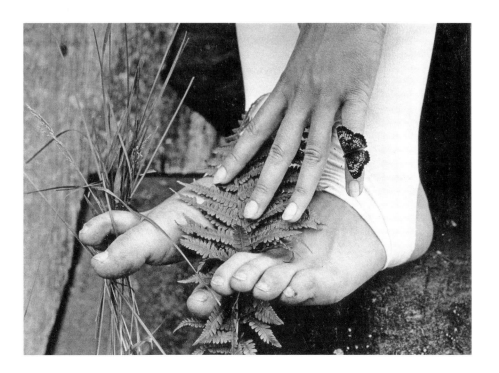

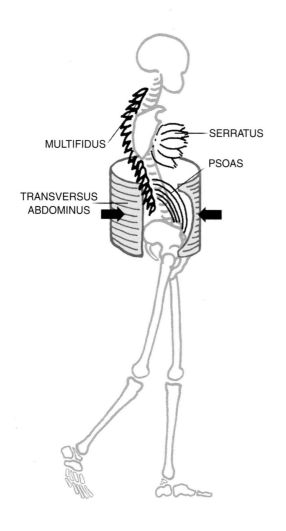

MULTIFIDUS

SERRATUS

PSOAS

TRANSVERSUS
ABDOMINUS

Fig. 11.22. *Major muscles of stabilization and locomotion.*
(Drawing by Susan Kress Hamilton.)

LORDOSIS AND CONTRALATERAL GAIT

Trunk stabilizers allow people to walk and run efficiently. The stability of the trunk adjusts to conserve the energy of gait, and the stability of the lumbar spine provides a counterforce against the actions of the hip flexors—the psoas muscles. With the trunk stabilized, the lumbar spine isn't pulled out of shape.

Gracovetsky shows that fish motion is the underlying engine of the spine and key for walking in human beings. A spine from the back wiggles side-to-side like a fish, as a person walks along. (To see this clearly, Gracovetsky invented a device called the Spinoscope that tracks the movement of the spine.) That side-to-side wiggle, lateral flexion, is turned into rotation by the nature of the spine's geometry.

Curved, flexible rods, when side-bent, produce torsion (twist) around their longitudinal axis. The spine is a curved, flexible rod. It has two lordoses (forward curves) and one main thoracic kyphosis (backward curve), as well as a sacral and occipital kyphosis. When you side-bend, the spine goes into states of torsion. In gait, there are counter-rotating groups of vertebrae in different sections of the spine. We felt the basic principle of this in our own bodies when we did Fish Spiral.

Watch a skillful runner and you will see opposed rotations of the upper and lower trunk. When the pelvis and lower spine rotates in one direction, the upper trunk will rotate the other direction. The spine is moving side to side, and it is being rotated. The pelvis takes the torsion from the spine and puts it into the legs. The rotary motion of the spine becomes forward and backward swing of the legs. The legs, in return, recycle the movement as the foot impacts and pushes off from the ground. That energy is delivered back to the spine as a whip-like force through the fascia and muscle tissue.

The set of opposing sagittal curves in the human spine are a key ingredient to successful upright posture and contralateral gait.

Sense impression in the hands and feet, articulation of the bones of the feet and lower legs, ample orientation to ground and space, responsive activity in the trunk-stabilizing muscles—all these are necessary for human walking and running.

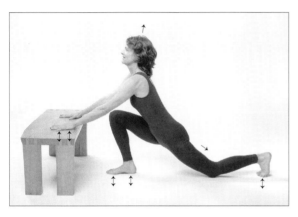

Fig. 11.23. *Flight of the Eagle.*
(All photographs of Flight of the Eagle, Part II by John Hession.)

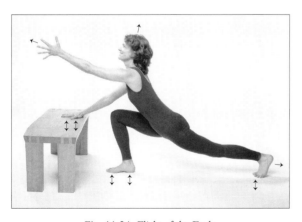

Fig. 11.24. *Flight of the Eagle.*

Exercise:
FLIGHT OF THE EAGLE, PART II

Once you feel comfortable with the first sequence described above, there are additional moves to Flight of the Eagle.

Start with your basic stance: feet on ground and hands on bench. Bring one foot forward close to the bench and place the other behind you so that your leg is extended fully with your toes on the ground and your heel in the air *(see Fig. 11.23)*. Reach forward and up with the hand on the same side as the extended leg. Reach behind you with your heel as you reach forward and up with your hand, all the while maintaining weight and stability with your other hand and foot on bench and floor. One side of your body is deeply lengthened in the front *(see Fig. 11.24)*.

Transfer your weight onto your stance foot and hand, and reach farther forward into the space in front of you. Your back leg stays straight and rises into the air and your outstretched hand and arm is in line with your extended back leg. This is a contralateral pose analogous to how you walk. You are supported by your hand on the bench and foot on the floor. You are also supported by your extended leg, the extended heel that reaches behind you, and your extended hand, also reaching into space. Your head is another limb reaching into space. Your body is supported by the array of vectors into space and ground. The body's coordination is effective but with little or no sense of effort. Support derives from sustained sensing of directions into space, and sustained loading into the hand and foot that are touching ground. There is support also from the other senses awake to the environment: sound, air on skin, peripheral vision, and smell. Using this support, reach your free hand toward the sky. As your hand reaches up, your body will rotate. Your head,

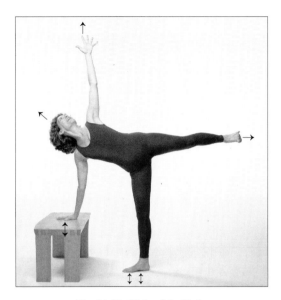

Fig. 11.25. *Flight of the Eagle.*

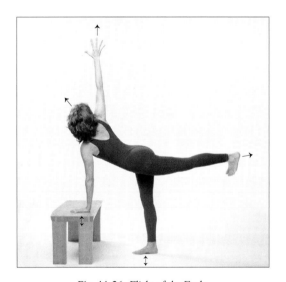

Fig. 11.26. *Flight of the Eagle.*

trunk, and extended leg will have all rotated to face the same side *(see Fig. 11.25).*

Next, transfer your support to the opposite hand and rotate the trunk, head, and leg to face the opposite direction. You are still supported by the original foot and leg. The extended leg has, however, rotated at the hip so the foot is facing the new side *(see Fig. 11.26).*

Standing on one leg can be made simpler and easier if you keep both hands on the bench while rotating your hip to one side and the other. Though less physically demanding, the challenge to sustain perception is similar, and the form is just as effective (see Figs. 11.27 and 11.28).

One Structural Integration client had this to say about Flight of the Eagle, Part II:

"It's amazing how the body calms down when you feel 'spiderman' suspension to space in different directions all around you. And every time you move you really have to start with the places touching the ground. It empowers you to move this way."

This man was in his late forties and had had back pain since he was seven years old, despite becoming an accomplished athlete. Using the Flight of the Eagle and other exercises, he was rehabilitating his back in a new way.

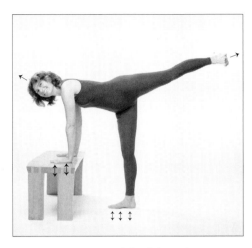

Fig. 11.27. *Flight of the Eagle.*

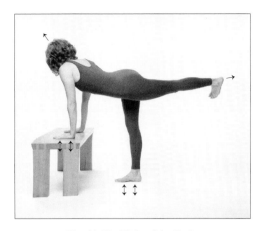

Fig. 11.28. *Flight of the Eagle.*

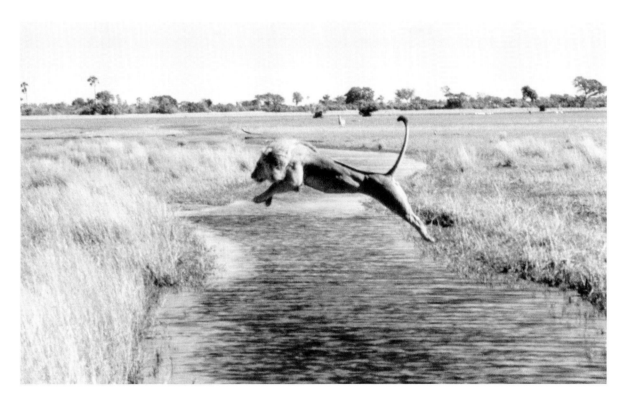

Fig. 11.29. Photograph by Peggy Keon.

FURTHER PERCEPTION-BASED EXERCISES

There are many ways to bring the sedentary human back into vitality, fluid movement, and stability. Begin any exercise with perception. Here are some more exercises to help you recover the joy of being an upright creature in gravity.

We work with relationship to ground and to space, and to some extent with relations between each other. We know something about beginning movement from a sense of weight and a sense of direction. We can also begin to move with an object. We can use imagination to shift the meaning of the object. By shifting the meaning of any object, we shift our relationship to that object;

this in turn changes how we move. We actually do this all the time.

When you walk toward someone to shake hands, or when the cashier offers you your change at the supermarket, you make a perception, an image, out of the person or object coming to you. Usually the way you treat others, whether they are things or people, is based on an image that is largely automatic.

Movement gives us the chance to be curious. If we can unlock the meaning of a simple object, something that isn't a big deal in our life story, then we can learn to unlock the meaning of other more challenging "objects" that show up in our life. Perhaps we can even apply this approach to our relationship stories, which tend to rule us. For now we will use a stick as our object. It will stand for the "other."

The stick we will use is either a $1^{3}/8$-inch diameter closet pole, cut about 30 inches long, or a similar size piece of sapling. The sapling can be of any hardwood species, and species that have a bumpy irregular bark are good choices. Irregular shape and texture can make it easier to feel.

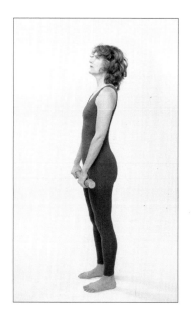
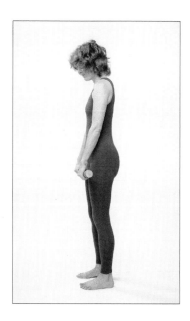

Exercise:
FOLDING, HOLDING A STICK

Stand with the stick held with both hands *(see Fig. 11.30)*. Your arms are hanging so the stick rests against your thighs, backs of hands facing out. Feel the floor touching your feet. Let the texture and temperature of the stick touch your hands. Imagine that the stick is quite heavy. Let your hands and the joints of your wrist, elbow, and shoulder register the imagined weight, as the stick pulls your arms down toward the floor. The weight of your stick helps the shoulder blades release fully from the spine. Allow your head to be pulled down, so your neck releases fully *(see Fig. 11.31)*. Your knees are drawn forward. Your heels feel the floor *(see Fig. 11.32)*. The stick pulls your hands down close to the floor and you are folded and bent forward *(see Fig. 11.33)*.

Now reverse the process. First, reestablish your feet on the floor. You push your feet into the floor to begin to unfold *(see Fig. 11.34)*. But you allow the stick to stay heavy. Use the pressure of your feet on the floor to uncurl the spine slowly toward an upright stance. Sustain the feeling of your feet pressing the floor, as you uncurl the spine slowly, segment by segment from the bottom up. As you uncurl, the knees reach forward, and the weight of your stick continues to keep your head and shoulders loaded.

Continue to let the exaggerated weight of the stick, and the pressure of the feet on the floor, uncurl the body toward upright stance. The knees continue to feel their forward vector as they extend. The head is the last thing to arrive. The spine has unfolded.

Rest for a moment; let your hands register the weight and texture of the stick. Let your feet load into the floor and feel the floor withstanding the load. Can you feel your shoulder girdle weighted even though the spine and the head are fully erect? The shoulders often engage to bring us upright. The heavy stick and our relationship to it can help prevent the shoulder muscles from pulling the spine up.

Figs. 11.30 and 11.31 at left; Figs. 11.32-11.34 below. *Folding, Holding a Stick* (All photographs by John Hession.)

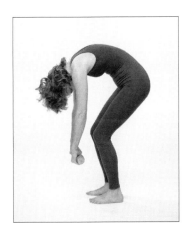
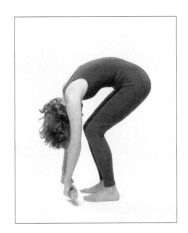
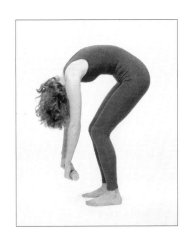

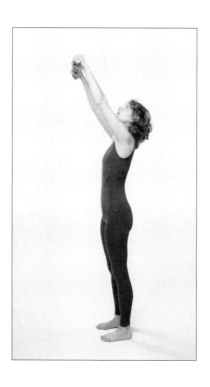

Notice the space around you. Imagine that the stick is getting very light, so light that it is buoyant. Like a large helium balloon, the stick can now lift your hands and arms. Feel the texture of the stick as you give it the power to lift your hands and arms upward until you are suspended from the stick, as though you were hanging from a chin-up bar. Keep your eyes on the stick. As the stick rises, continue to feel your feet on the floor. Feel the weight shift from heel to toes. Let your toes spread and lengthen with the shift of balance in your whole body. As you allow the toes to be pressed into the floor, you are allowing the stick to lengthen the front of your body in space *(see Figs. 11.35 and 11.36).*

Can you notice space all around you when you move? Can you notice the space beside you, above you, and behind you, as well as in front of you? Can you notice the buoyant stick still holding your arms high? Can you feel your toes press and reach forward to offer support?

When you are ready, allow the stick to become heavy, drawing your hands and arms down toward the floor. Let weight come back into your heels and begin the folding process as before.

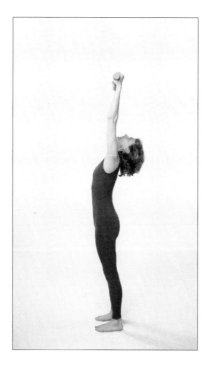

Figs. 11.35 and 11.36. *The Buoyant Stick.*
(Photographs by John Hession.)

Exercise:
SITTING UP WITH A STICK

Sitting up with a stick in your hands is a mirror for your capacity to stay related to ground, space, and object. Take care to work on perception rather than effort with muscles.

Lie on your back with your legs straight. The stick is held in your hands and lies on your belly or chest. Notice the floor touching you. Notice the sky or ceiling above. You are first a child of Heaven and Earth before you do any movement.

Let the texture of the stick speak to your hands. Feel the mass of it. Imagine the stick becomes buoyant and rises, taking your hands with it into the space above you *(see Fig. 11.37)*. When the stick has lifted your hands and arms, allow the shoulder blades to be brought forward on your rib cage. Your shoulder girdle is lifted aloft while your spine is resting on the floor.

Feel your legs and heels contact the floor as you imagine the stick gaining even greater lift. The stick lifts you farther as you hang from it and your spine rises with the lifting shoulder girdle *(see Figs. 11.38 and 11.39)*. The head momentarily back-bends on the neck due to its weight, but then even the head is pulled aloft, and the chest, upper spine, and head are supported by the power of the stick. The belly is relatively soft. The sit-up happens without engagement of the rectus chain of muscles, or only a little and late in the process *(see Figs. 11.40 and 11.41)*.

The stick teaches you to find pre-movement that releases your spine. The tonic chain of back muscles first lengthens, allowing your body to rise off the ground freely. Brakes let go before gas pedal is applied. The stick teaches you to move by finding sense impression, weight, and space orientation, and by allowing an object to affect you. You receive object impression so that your

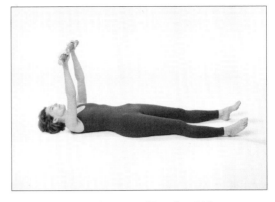

Fig. 11.37. *Sitting Up with a Stick.*
(All photographs by John Hession.)

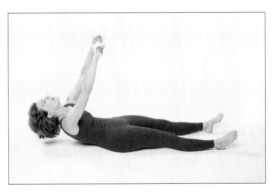

Fig. 11.38. *Sitting Up with a Stick.*

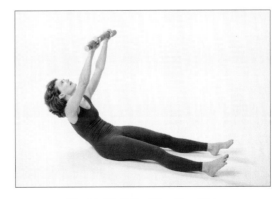

Fig. 11.39. *Sitting Up with a Stick.*

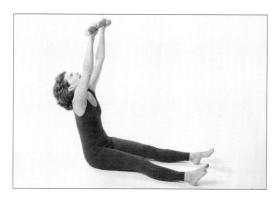

Fig. 11.40. *Sitting Up with a Stick.*

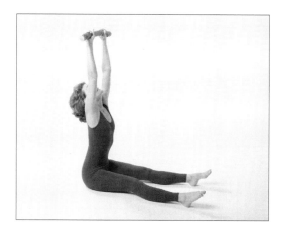

Fig. 11.41. *Sitting Up with a Stick.*

You can rehabilitate core stabilization and emphasize hands and feet, space, and weight using elastic therapy bands. You need a piece of medium- or heavy-rated band, about 7 feet long, and a fixed object on the wall or floor to tie it to. To do these exercises, tie your 7-foot band into a loop.

movement is unbound, not inhibited by thoughts of how to do it

A partner makes this exercise easier. One person stands stands above, straddling his or her partner at about waist level, and slowly lifts the stick. The other, on the floor, allows the stick to help the back release and go forward. The challenge is the same: Allow the sense impression in the hand, the sense of the stick, and the broad orientation to ground and space to remind the body to move naturally.

Attach the elastic band to a fixed point on the floor or on the wall just above the floor. Face toward the band and loop it around your ankle. Your pre-movement starts by feeling the ground under your feet and then feeling the standing foot become large and planted in the floor. How deeply can you connect the standing leg into the ground below you? As you drop weight and press into the planted foot, begin to notice your head in space. How omni-directionally can your skull feel space? How tall and distant is your sense of horizon?

Increase the pressure of the standing (un-banded) foot and amplify the sense of space around your head until your opposite hip and leg lift slightly, and your banded foot hovers just off the floor. Refresh the sense of down in your standing foot and up and out in your head and peripheral vision. Then move your banded foot and leg behind you, as you raise your hand and arm forward on the same side.

Only a short range of motion is necessary. You will feel the success of this exercise when you feel the trunk lengthen and stabilize itself. You will feel the shift in your whole body as a result of what you do with your sense of ground and space. The band gives you a more tangible feed-back to the extending leg, but you strengthen something more important than muscle power. You strengthen the ability of the body to recruit muscles correctly. Your job is to feel sense impression in the hands and feet and to orient yourself to "spiderman" suspension. Notice the calm that comes from being supported by imaginary filaments between your body and the potent space around you.

The value of this exercise is multi-fold. You are teaching your body to recruit transversus abdominus and multifidus muscles to stabilize your trunk against a load. You are stimulating your body to stabilize efficiently at the sacroiliac joint. This exercise also stimulates contralateral gait, as does the following exercise.

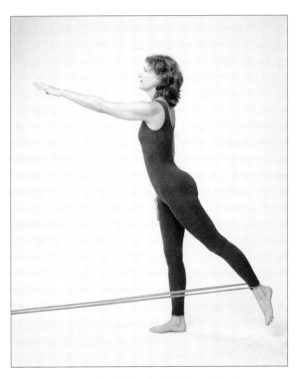

Fig. 11.42. *Arabesque with Therapy Band.*
(Photograph by John Hession.)

Exercise:
SHOT PUT WITH THERAPY BAND

The band can be attached to object or wall at the same level as in the previous exercise or it can be anywhere between floor and chest height. Stand with your side to the band and grasp the band with the hand on the side closest to the band. Your feet are in a wide stance. Your pre-movement involves finding your feet and their relation to the ground. The foot on the band side of your body can pivot and roll onto the toes. The other foot should stay planted. Both feet should feel large and planted as you start. Allow your knees to bend so you are a little crouched, gathering the energy of an animal preparing to pounce *(see Fig. 11.43)*.

Your head should notice omni-directional space. Notice the horizon opposite the wall or attachment point of your band. The hand with the band crosses over your body and projects the band toward the horizon, while the back foot pivots and comes onto the toes. You might feel a two-directional span between your hand and the toes of your back foot *(see Fig. 11.44)*.

One student reported after doing the shot put with band:

> *"I felt wild and powerful. It helped me feel like I was projecting something far into the distance. After establishing my feet, the sense of the far horizon unleashed a rush of energy and movement."*

The Shot Put exercise is a torsion exercise—torsion with hands and feet engaged. The crouch and the twist stimulate action in the transversus abdominus and internal oblique. The reach and projection of the hand stimulate action in the serratus anterior, and the rhomboids lengthen. The body has the opportunity to feel a strong contralateral gesture that rehabilitates contralateral gait.

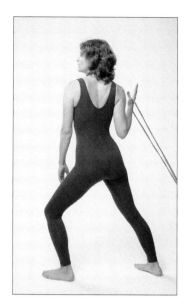

Fig. 11.43. *Shot Put with Therapy Band.* (Photograph by John Hession.)

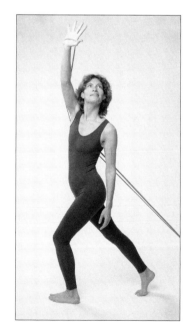

Fig. 11.44. *Shot Put with Therapy Band.* (Photograph by John Hession.)

No exercise alone can restore natural strength, flow, and health. No metaphor or clever inspiration lifts us out of our habits of perception, coordination, and meaning. We try some things and in the process we improve our odds for something new to occur, perhaps during an exercise, or sometimes as we allow ourselves to openly attend. In moments of open attention we may notice what has been aroused by the exercises, by the inquiry associated with them.

The evolutionary story is an invitation for you to innovate. Find out what is true for you, and find out what is occurring as sensation. Explore the potency of space and weight, of imagined arrows of direction. Feel sense impression in your hands and feet, and skin, each time freshly.

Find out if it is possible for your body to move freely and without a sense of effort.

NOTES FOR TEACHERS AND BODY THERAPISTS

Issues of lordosis, its development, our cultural attitude toward it, and ways in which regulation of lordosis can become congruent with natural function are controversial. This is an exciting time to work with these issues. New research about back pain, combined with Godard's tonic function model, makes it possible to better answer our clients'/students' questions about back stability. We want people to look critically at every therapy or movement instruction they receive.

The exercises in this chapter are different from those in preceding chapters in a number of ways. These explorations have a different flavor partly because they are adaptations of work that Godard has presented in his classes for Structural Integrators. They bear his imprint. We are bringing our work into upright situations that challenge us as we might be challenged in daily life, physically as well as psychologically. The last three exercises teach us about sustaining broad orientation, bi-directionality of line, when confronting relational challenges.

We assume that at this point in the book, students have gained some anatomical knowledge and understand the story of spinal movement that unfolds in the preceding chapters. We assume some familiarity with moving from perception. These exercises can be taught to clients or students who might have less interest or patience to delve deeply into the creature story. However, to successfully teach these exercises perceptually, one must embody them oneself.

Even then, the value of doing something like Flight of the Eagle will not be immediately obvious to most students. How do we communicate its value? How do we excite people to experiment? Each of us will find our own relationship to the work. It can be helpful to use simple metaphors that illustrate the magic of tonic function. In the Bibliography we list some articles about tonic function theory that might help fill out your knowledge of this approach.

The topic of lordosis is usually interesting to anyone who has done movement. We think it is a good idea to name the topics that are likely to be controversial and invite students to share their stories at the outset. After the teacher has presented his or her view about back health and spinal regulation, students may temporarily discount their personal experiences.

Stabilization of the spine is an integrated system event. We name some of the muscles that are useful to think about. It is helpful to differentiate the layers of the belly wall and distinguish their function. We teach this anatomy to our clients and students because we believe it empowers people to know certain aspects of anatomy, especially when attending yoga classes, martial arts classes, or becoming a patient in the medical system.

Anatomy can be empowering. Anatomy can also be problematic. Thinking about muscles during movement tends to reduce integrated function. Thinking about muscles is a distraction from what turns on our system of core integrity and coordination. The dilemma for a movement teacher is to use the anatomy in useful ways and at the same time help students to let go of the biomechanical model when they are learning a new movement.

The same dilemma applies in mentioning a concept such as contralateral gait. Contralateral gait is a concept that can easily lead to "concocted" movement. Contralateral, homolateral, homologous—these are all terms that need to be taught with care. Structural integration helps liberate contralateral gait but this natural aspect of walking emerges when inhibition is released, when perception releases the habit patterns that get in the way.[4] The evolutionary sequence establishes experiences and skills that make concepts like contralateral gait more digestible.

WORKING WITH "OTHER"

Working with the sense of "other" offers students an opportunity to change perception. As mentioned before, this is also an opportunity to work with relational politics. We must keep "other" from becoming another place of confusion.

How do we work with building a sense of other? We allow our senses to be touched by the world. We *think* we live with a strong sense of other already. Is this true? Don't we want to free ourselves from a sense of self and other? These are great questions for discussion in movement study.

We suggest that most of us have very little *sense* of other. We live with a powerful *story* about other. We have an image or thoughts about other and others. For example, one has stories about parents, partners, children, co-workers. But this just means we are fused to all these "outside" objects. A strong story about a person or object typically ensures that we will have no functional articulation when we move in relation to the object. When we begin to move, our movement will involve co-contraction, fusing of the girdles with the spine as long as the story of other dominates our awareness.

Why do stories of other block flow of movement? Our stories about the other are based on an attempt to master the other. In this manner we cope with our limited or lack of power in relating to the world. We cope by making a story. Our story gives us a way of organizing our experience. I remember an event and I picture the event or talk to myself about the event. As I rehearse my history, I reinforce the habit patterns in my muscles. My muscles had a response to mastering a situation. This response lives on as a habit of body defenses I develop to ensure that I will be able to handle the next encounter.

For example, if I have had difficulty or embarrassment in throwing a ball, how might this illustrate my relationship to other? Perhaps I was taught to throw by my older brother. The first throw was a naïve experiment. I watched my brother's throw and then attempted to imitate his. On my first try I let go of the ball too soon and it fell near my feet. I wanted to do better. Perhaps my brother, having a sincere desire to help, said, "Don't let go of the ball!" This time I held on to the ball tightly and used muscles in my legs and arms and neck to make sure that the ball would not be released too early. I never again lost control of the ball. I "mastered" the ball with my whole body.

However, now the story of the ball, my hand and shoulder girdle, and the ball itself are all glued together as one thing. When I throw the ball as an adult, the story may not have changed. A body therapist, dance coach, or movement teacher will easily observe the tension, the shortening of my neck, the restraint in my rhomboid (and other) muscles when I throw a ball. There is no other, because the story of other ensures that I will continue to reenact what I have always done in the unconscious wish to never drop the ball prematurely again! How do I rehabilitate this?

I need to be free of the pattern of mastering, the defense against failure. Rather than working this in an explicitly psychological way, we can work with movement, imagination, and sensation. We can, through sense impression, inhibit the inhibition, as Godard has phrased it. We can learn to calm the forces of defense against failure. In all our perceptual work we have invited happy accidents, innovative discoveries in which the brakes that hold back natural movement are released. Here we name the sense of other. It is dramatic to start with an image of other and replace it with sustained sensory impression of the thing itself, in sensation.

Sensation in the moment of perception liberates us from the story of other by replacing the story with something that, moment to moment, is actually happening. We build a sense of other when we learn to sustain sense impression. To be touched by the other is not enough. To build a sense of other we must take in sense impression of the object that represents other, and simultaneously maintain a broad orientation to space and weight. Then, other can provide the element of articulation, of appropriate differentiation between the self and other.

Differentiated sensory orientation frees our movement (and consciousness) from many stories. We do not need to defend from being touched by the world. A person, who is adequately and richly oriented to space and weight, and to sense impression of other, will move with greater flow.

NOTES FOR TEACHERS AND BODY THERAPISTS ON TONIC FUNCTION AND SPINAL STABILIZATION

We live in a time when core stabilization enjoys a wave of popularity in the fitness world. Carolyn Richardson's work on segmental stabilization is one resource from which you can find research that supports a fresh look at what makes a healthy back.[5] Tonic function emphasizes the use of perception to change coordination. Scientific research shows that the recruitment of muscles such as transversus abdominus and multifidus must be retaught, that the coordination must be relearned for subjects with back pain. However, researchers have only begun to consider how to teach this to people.[6,7] Tonic function is an attempt to answer the question, "What helps people learn healthy coordination?"

We want to find out what prevents healthy movement. We want to find movement where the muscles that compress the spine can let go, where the transversus abdominus and multifidus lengthen the trunk at the beginning of the movement. We want to teach people how it feels to stabilize the core without thinking about the core.

Gracovetsky's book *The Spinal Engine*[8] is worth tracking down because it includes an exhaustive study of how the spine is able to handle loads. His diagrams help us understand how the core stabilizers function. He demonstrates that only the multifidus group has the fiber angles and attachment positions to adequately act as a true erector of the spine. The larger group of muscles typically referred to as erector spinae acts largely to side-bend the trunk rather than erect it.

Gracovetsky also demonstrates the manner in which the transverses abdominus supports the trunk like a corset and specifically reinforces the posterior ligaments of the lumbar spine. The transversus and multifidus, as part of the posterior fascial net, supply counterforces to the anterior force supplied by the psoas on the lumbar vertebrae.

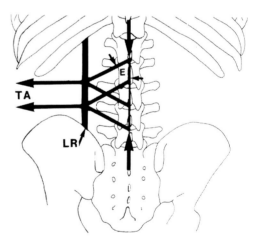

Fig. 11.45. *The transversus abdominus acts to tense fascia and ligaments of the lumbar spine, stabilizing the spine.* (Reproduced with kind permission from Serge Gracovetsky.)

The physics of contralateral gait are also described in a separate paper by Gracovetsky.[9] His model can be reduced to some basic observations about human locomotive function. These are summarized below.

During walking and running, people are free to allow the shoulder girdle and upper trunk to freely counter-rotate the lower trunk and pelvis. When we start to walk forward, the story gets more complex. Fish body motion of the spine is converted into rotation of the pelvis so we can walk. This walk happens even in the absence of legs. Gracovetsky had a patient born without legs. This patient's spine and pelvis move in the same way as people walking on their two legs.

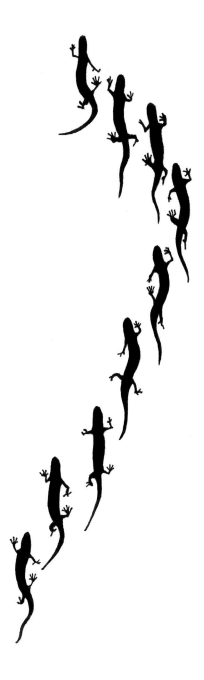

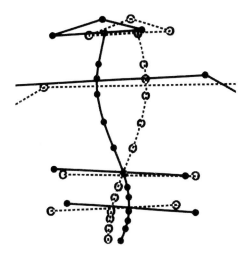

Fig. 11.46 right. *The locomotion cycle of the newt shows fish motion with limbs.* (Redrawn with kind permission from Serge Gracovetsky.)

Fig. 11.47 above. *The Spinoscope uses LEDs to show the fish motion of human subjects from the back during walking. The LEDs indicate the positions of spine processes. Notice the two distinct side-bends occurring. The lumbar and thoracic side-bends exchange roles from gait-moment to gait-moment. Here, the solid line represents one moment; the dotted line represents the next moment.*
(Reproduced with kind permission from Serge Gracovetsky.)

To enable the spine to rotate and counter-rotate, to allow the upper trunk and shoulder girdle to receive, store, and return the rotational energy initiated as the spine side-bends, the spine must reverse its rotation at some point near the bottom of the thoracic. The two sides of the spine are alternately lengthening in the front and the back in a sequential wave of movement that corresponds to the flexion and extension of the hip.

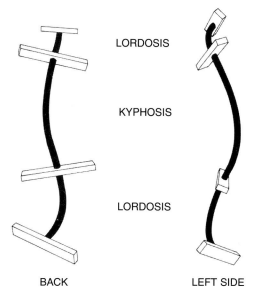

LORDOSIS

KYPHOSIS

LORDOSIS

BACK   LEFT SIDE

Fig. 11.48. *The human spine rotates and counter-rotates through its curves, leaving the head to face forward.* (Reproduced with kind permission from Serge Gracovetsky.)

Energy is conserved in a number of ways. The force of the foot landing on the heel transmits back up the leg and into the spine where it amplifies the rotation and side-bending. The force of the toes bending before push-off helps release the front of the hip and the front surface of the trunk on that side. The arms and shoulders act as a horizontal flywheel that receives and delivers back the rotary force of the trunk.

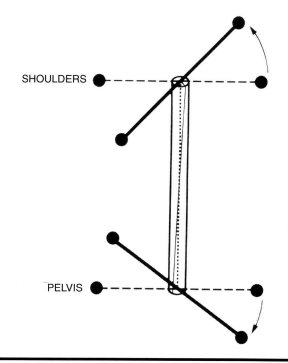

SHOULDERS

PELVIS

Fig. 11.49. *The upright human spine is an efficient oscillating system in which energy of rotation is exchanged from lower movement to upper, and vice versa.* (Reproduced with kind permission from Serge Gracovetsky.)

The shoulders are not a good way to hold up the chest, neck, and head. If rhomboids work to hold up the upper spine, they will impede the flow of spinal movement in walking. When we allow the stick to hold the shoulders down through a sense of weight, and use orientation to find length and elongation of the spine, we remove an impediment to flow in walking. When we walk, the hands can be alive with their sense of weight and the air around them. The head is oriented broadly to sky. These perceptions provide support. The shoulders can then abstain from potential mischief.

Teaching students to see and embody the sense of contralateral gait involves both biomechanical explanation and movement explorations. When we alternate our moving and meaning-making, we slowly awaken the natural coordinative impulses that serve our species not only in walking but in traditional forms of human work and play. Scything a field, sowing seed, poling or paddling a boat, hauling nets or ropes, throwing a ball or spear—in each activity we operate our contralateral mechanism. In all these activities, and others, the stabilizers of the trunk, transversus abdominus and multifidus in the lower trunk and serratus anterior in the upper trunk, are in continuous use.

Fig. 11.50. *"Humans" (detail of Indonesian textile).*

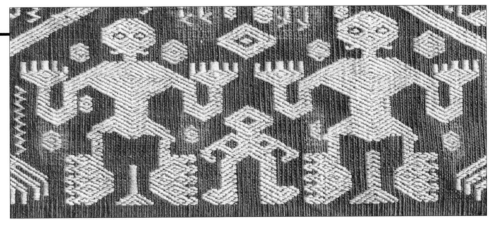

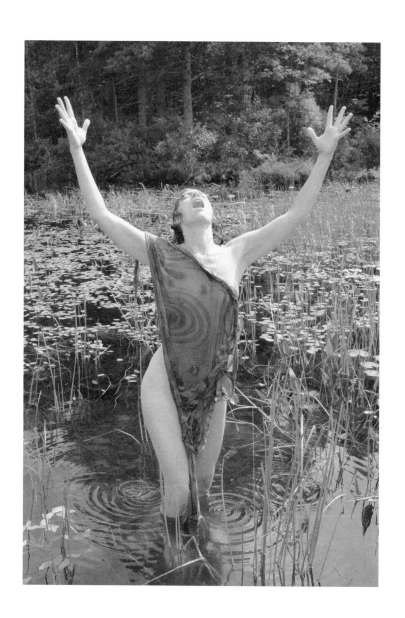

"Every day [and each moment] we must rebuild the world; we must rebuild ground and space."

HUBERT GODARD

POURING INTO THE LIMBS, FEELING BIFURCATION [1]— AN EXPLORATION TO STAND AND MEET THE WORLD.

Roll your body on the floor to revive the sense of skin, the sense of flow in omni-directional awareness. As you roll, pour your fluid contents back and forth until you feel soft. Roll yourself onto your hands and feet until you are completely poured into your limbs and you feel the impression of the ground flowing back into your hands and feet.

Orient your head and tail with two directions into space, making sure you feel the fluid weight you have established in your whole body. There is a moment one can enjoy the bifurcation of the limbs off of the spine into the hands and feet. One may feel that the body is only hands and feet and spine, alive to context.

Walk the hands toward the feet, deeply flexing in your hip, knee, and ankle. Slowly transfer weight into your legs. Begin pouring into your feet and legs, allowing articulation in the sacroiliac joint and pubic symphysis, each of these a bifurcation. Feel the spine erecting from your contact with Earth. Allow the shoulder girdles to slide freely, and the spine to flow through it. Sense bifurcation where the clavicles meet the sternum. Give your eyes, ears, nose, and mouth time to touch and be touched by the world. Notice presence in your weighted fluid body. Feel alive to space.

Lift the arms. Before doing so, let the feet receive and deliver the weight of the arms to the ground with an extra squirt. Accelerate the sense of pouring from the arms into the torso and into the legs. Let the hands sense the space in front of the gut body. Let the gut body feel weight and let it orient to the environment, gently. Allow the arms to rise until they are above the head. Slowly rotate the palms outward, feeling the air, noticing the space. Then lower the arms, caressing the air as they come down, and feel your feet touching the ground at the same time. How do you meet the world in this moment?

HOW TO USE THIS BOOK

What's the most important thing to focus on as you do these exercises? It's not about deifying the animals and it's not about "getting it right." The most important point is experimentation and widening perception to what is possible. Keep the following things in mind as you explore. Find out how you prepare to move. Find out about how your body orients itself, through meaning, through sense of weight and space. Begin to enlarge your vocabulary of sensation, slowing down your perception of what is sensed. Find out what it means to build a sense of "other."

The point of doing these exercises is to create a way of moving and being that opens perception, so habitual ways of operating are discovered and replaced with awareness. It is in this place of awareness that innovation can be born and the inquiry into what it means to be alive, in a human body, gets interesting.

Movement flow is our natural birthright. What prevents it? Traditional movement forms offer us a record of human invention. But form doesn't guarantee flow. In fact, form may inhibit flow. Questioning form to revive flow is a creative process that offers the chance to do something completely new. Enjoy the pleasure of unique moments of discovery.

APPENDIX A: Rolf and Godard

Born in 1895, IDA P. ROLF was a biochemist who created a new way to treat musculoskeletal problems and improve posture. Her protocol, Structural Integration, is a provocative way of shifting the underlying causes of the muscle conflict problem. Rolf also proposed that this approach could be part of an inquiry into human evolution. Her protocol got a reputation for making dramatic changes in her clients through manipulation of fascia. Fascia, Rolf claimed, could be reshaped through deep strategic manipulation using a series of approximately ten sessions.

Rolf's work became popular in the 1960s during the emergence of the "human potential movement," something that was particularly associated with Esalen Institute in Big Sur, California. Later, Rolf founded the Rolf Institute, which still teaches her work and investigates possibilities for improving human movement and function.

HUBERT GODARD represents a second generation of Structural Integration thinking. Like Rolf, he was born to innovate the field of somatic inquiry.

Godard grew up in France, the son of a farmer; he went to various boarding schools and excelled in handball and fencing. He was trained as a chemist and eventually became one of the youngest people to be licensed to perform metallurgy for the recovery of gold in industrial waste.

In his early twenties Godard also became fascinated with dance, the quality of human movement through space, and the sense of lift and flight he observed in the performers. Within a few years he was dancing seriously. But he suffered damage to his knee because dance forms and the architecture of his body were not congruent. Godard's proclivity for mechanics and problem solving, together with his knack for meeting the right people at the right time, led him to osteopathy and the world of soft tissue and bony manipulation, which he mastered in short order.

Godard was invited to chair a new department at the University of Paris that would organize and improve dance instruction in France.

Godard trained in Ida Rolf's method of Structural Integration. This gave Godard a sense that life in and out of the dance studio weren't separate. It also confirmed a vision of movement and relationship to gravity that integrated all his other studies in osteopathy, Feldenkrais method, Alexander technique, Mézières method, classical dance, and even psychoanalysis. Gravity became the unifying principle that tied psychology, body therapy, and the aesthetics of movement together.

Godard started teaching structural integrators around 1990. Since then, he has taught worldwide, and continues to direct research primarily at a cancer research institute in Milan, Italy.

We, the authors, are among the fortunate who have worked with Godard. This book, as well as articles we have on our web site, attempts to translate the tonic function approach into practical tools and explanations for the student of movement and bodywork.

F. M. ALEXANDER (1869–1955) was an Australian actor who studied how to unlock habits of movement, beginning with his own body's vocal constrictions. We learn to unlock our movements at a fundamental level, through orientation to space, and before our goal-oriented mind is engaged. His contributions are carried on in the work known as Alexander Technique.

MOSHE FELDENKRAIS (1904–1984) was a European physicist, engineer, and martial artist. Through analysis and personal experimentation he created a vast catalog of perceptual interventions for unlocking movement habit and encouraging movement innovation. His contributions are carried on in the work known as Feldenkrais Method.

FRANÇOISE MÉZIÈRES (1909–1991) was a French physiotherapist and anatomy and physiology teacher who discovered that the body's movement control must be addressed through its tonic system, through the chains of muscles that govern automatic postural response. Her work has been described partially in English by Therese Bertherat in the book *The Body Has Its Reasons: Self Awareness Through Conscious Movement*.

EMILIE CONRAD started Continuum in 1967 and continues to teach this provocative approach to rediscovering the fundamental impulses and waves within the human body. Conrad's contribution is especially significant as she creates new approaches to rehabilitation, most notably spinal cord injury, by working with unusual primitive movements reminiscent of cells, sea creatures, and mythic images.

SUSAN HARPER collaborated with Emilie Conrad in the development of Continuum and now teaches under the title Continuum Montage. Harper trains bodyworkers and therapists; she leads inquiry into what broad skills and resources allow us to stay present in challenging and novel circumstances.

PETER LEVINE is a neuropsychologist, Rolfer, and inventor of a technique he calls Somatic Experiencing. Somatic Experiencing (SE) assists people who have suffered shock and trauma to reestablish self-regulation. Levine's work is based on observations of mammals surviving challenges in the wild. He uses the natural world to find answers to our human problems. His work is carried on by the Foundation for Human Enrichment.

BONNIE BAINBRIDGE COHEN made discoveries about developmental movement in children and perceptual strategies for children dealing with severe delays. She founded the School for Body Mind Centering.

WENDY PALMER is an Aikido teacher who brings the dynamics of perceptual balance to the arena of relational challenge. She speaks to the underlying intelligence of our movement through perception and orientation.

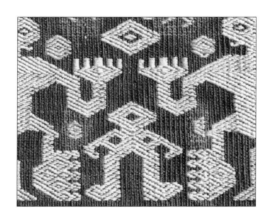

BIBLIOGRAPHY AND RESOURCES
FOR THE STUDY OF EVOLUTION, MOVEMENT SCIENCE, AND
PERCEPTUAL APPROACHES TO MOVEMENT AND CONSCIOUSNESS

Bertherat, T., *The Body Has Its Reasons: Self-Awareness Through Conscious Movement*. Rochester, Vermont: Healing Arts Press, 1989.

Blakeslee, S., "Complex and Hidden Brain in Gut Makes Stomachaches and Butterflies." *New York Times*, 23 January 1996, sec. C1.

Blechshmidt, E., *The Ontogenetic Basis of Human Anatomy: A Biodynamic Approach to Development from Conception to Birth*. Berkeley: North Atlantic Books, 2004.

Bond, M., *Balancing Your Body*. Rochester, Vermont: Healing Arts Press, 1996.

Borg, S., *The Migraine Puzzle*. Burlington, Vermont: Resonant Kinesiology Media Productions, 1993.

Borg, S., in collaboration with McHose, C., and Nesson, R., *Sing Your Body*. Burlington, Vermont: Resonant Kinesiology Media Productions, 1993.

Brown, H., "The Other Brain, the One with Butterflies, Also Deals with Many Woes." *New York Times*, 23 August 2005, sec. D5.

Buchsbaum, R., Buchsbaum, M., Pearse, V., and Pearse, J., *Animals Without Backbones: An Introduction to the Invertebrates*, Third Edition. Chicago: University of Chicago Press, 1987.

Burnett, N., and Matsen, B., *The Shape of Life*. Monterey, Calif.: Monterey Bay Aquarium Press, 2002.

Calais-Germain, B., *Anatomy of Movement*. Seattle: Eastland Press, 1993.

Caspari, M., "The Functional Rationale of the Recipe." *2005 IASI Yearbook*, pp. 51–78. Missoula, Montana: IASI, 2005.

Clarke, B., *Eyewitness Books: Amphibian*. New York: Alfred A. Knopf, 1993.

Clemente, C., *Anatomy: A Regional Atlas of the Human Body*. Baltimore and Munich: Urban and Schwarzenberg, 1987.

Cohen, B. B., *Sensing, Feeling, Action: The Experiential Anatomy of Body-Mind Centering*. Northampton, Mass.: Contact Editions, 1993.

Frank, K., "Flight of the Eagle—Self Care for Structural Integration Clients." *2005 IASI Yearbook*, pp. 44–50. Missoula, Mont.: IASI, 2005.

Frank, K., "Gravity Orientation as the Basis for Structural Integration." *Heller Work Newsletter*, Spring 1994, pp. 16–18. Seattle: Hellerwork Association.

Frank, K., "The Relationship of Contralateral Gait and the Tonic Function Model of Structural Integration." *Journal of Structural Integration*, Dec. 2003, pp. 17–21. Boulder: Rolf Institute.

Frank, K., "Seeing the Ground of a Movement: Tonic Function and the Fencing Bear." *2004 IASI Yearbook*, pp. 103–104. Missoula, Mont.: IASI, 2004.

Frank, K., "Stuart Hameroff's Theories Regarding Microtubules as the Seat of Consciousness." *Rolf Lines*, Nov. 1998, pp. 38–40. Boulder: Rolf Institute.

Frank, K., "Tonic Function—A Gravity Response Model for Rolfing® Structural and Movement Integration." *Rolf Lines*, March 1995, pp. 12–20. Boulder: Rolf Institute.

Frank, K., "Wave Motion and the Fluid Matrix." *Convergence Magazine*, 1995, pp. 20–23. Concord, N.H.: Virginia Slayton.

Frank, K., "Working with Coordinative Structure, Tonic Function and Contralateral Gait." *Journal of Structural Integration,* Spring 2004. Boulder: Rolf Institute.

Franklin, E., *Dynamic Alignment through Imagery*, Champaign, Il: Human Kinetics, 1996.

Gershon, M., *The Second Brain: A Groundbreaking New Understanding of Nervous Disorders of the Stomach and Intestine.* New York: Harper Collins, 1999.

Godard, H., "Reading the Body in Dance," *Rolf Lines*, Oct. 1994, pp. 37–42. Boulder: Rolf Institute.

Goldfield, E., *Emergent Forms: Origins and Early Development of Human Action and Perception.* New York: Oxford University Press, 1995.

Gould, S. J., *The Book of Life: An Illustrated History of the Evolution of Life on Earth.* New York: W. W. Norton & Co., 1993.

Gracovetsky, S., "Analysis and Integration of Gait in Relation to Lumbo Pelvic Pain." *4th Interdisciplinary Congress on Low Back and Pelvic Pain.* Montreal, November 2001.

Gracovetsky, S., *The Spinal Engine.* Wien and New York: Springer-Verlag, 1988.

Grossinger, R., *Embryogenesis.* Berkeley: North Atlantic Books, 1986.

Haeckel, E., *Art Forms in Nature.* Mineola, N.Y.: Dover Press, 1974.

Johnson, J., and Gray, E., *Skeletons: An Inside Look at Animals.* Pleasantville, N.Y.: Readers Digest Association, Inc., 1994.

Jones, L., *Strain and Counterstrain.* Newark, Ohio: The American Academy of Osteopathy, 1981.

Juhan, D., *Job's Body.* Barrytown, N.Y.: Station Hill Press, 1987.

Kapandji, I. A., *The Physiology of the Joints, Vol. 1, Upper Limb.* New York: Churchill Livingstone, 1982.

Kapandji, I. A., *The Physiology of the Joints, Vol. 2, Lower Limb.* New York: Churchill Livingstone, 1987.

Kapandji, I. A., *The Physiology of the Joints, Vol. 3, The Trunk and the Vertebral Column.* New York: Churchill Livingstone, 1974.

Lee, D., "An Integrated Model of Joint Function and Its Clinical Application." *4th Interdisciplinary Congress on Low Back and Pelvic Pain*. Montreal, November 2001.

Levine, P., *Waking the Tiger.* Berkeley: North Atlantic Books, 1997.

Llinas, R. R., *I of the Vortex: From Neurons to Self.* Cambridge: MIT Press, 2001.

Maitland, J., *Spacious Body.* Berkeley: North Atlantic Books, 1995.

Margulis, L., and Sagan, D., *What Is Life?* New York: Simon and Schuster, 1993.

McCarthy, C., *Eyewitness Books: Reptile.* New York: Alfred A. Knopf, 1991.

McHose, C., and Frank, K., "The Evolutionary Sequence: A Model for an Integrative Approach to Movement Study." *Rolf Lines,* May 1998, pp. 37–49. Boulder: Rolf Institute.

Myers, T., *Anatomy Trains: Myofascial Meridians for Manual and Movement Therapists.* New York: Churchill Livingstone, 2001.

Netter, F., *Atlas of Human Anatomy.* Summit, N.J.: Ciba-Geigy Corporation, 1989.

Newbert, C., *Within a Rainbow Sea.* Hillsboro, Oregon: Beyond Words Publishing, 1984.

Newbert, C., and Wilms, B., *In a Sea of Dreams.* San Antonio, Texas: Fourth Day Publishing, 1994.

Newton, A., "Basic Concepts in the Work of Hubert Godard." *Rolf Lines*, March 1995, pp. 32–42. Boulder: Rolf Institute.

Newton, A., "Breathing in the Gravity Field." *Rolf Lines,* Fall 1997, pp-27–35. Boulder: Rolf Institute.

Newton, A., "Core Stabilization, Core Coordination." *Journal of Structural Integration*, Dec. 2003, pp. 11–16. Boulder: Rolf Institute.

Newton, A., "Gracovetsky and Walking." *Journal of Structural Integration*, Feb. 2003, pp. 4–8. Boulder: Rolf Institute.

Newton, A., "An Interview with Hubert Godard." *Rolf Lines,* Winter, 1992, pp. 42–49. Boulder: Rolf Institute.

Newton, A., "New Conceptions of Breathing Anatomy and Biomechanics." *Rolf Lines,* Winter 1998, pp. 29–37. Boulder: Rolf Institute.

Newton, A., "Posture and Gravity." *Rolf Lines*, April 1998, pp. 35–38. Boulder: Rolf Institute.

Ni, H., *I-Ching: The Book of Changes and the Unchanging Truth.* Santa Monica: Sevenstar Communications, Inc., 1983.

Ohlgren, G., and Clark, D., "Natural Walking." *Rolf Lines*, March 1995, pp. 21–29. Boulder: Rolf Institute.

Olsen, A., *Body and Earth.* Hanover, N.H.: University Press of New England, 2002.

Olsen, A., in collaboration with McHose, C., *Bodystories: A Guide to Experiential Anatomy.* Barrytown, N.Y.: Station-Hill Openings, 1991.

Oschman, J., *Energy Medicine in Therapeutics and Human Performance.* New York: Butterworth and Heinemann, 2003.

Oschman, J., and Oschman, N., *Readings on the Scientific Basis of Bodywork,* Vol II. Dover, N.H.: 1995.

Packer, T., *Seeing Without Knowing.* Springwater, N.Y.: Springwater Center, 1983.

Packer, T., *The Wonder of Presence.* Boston: Shambhala, 2002.

Packer, T., *The Work of This Moment.* Springwater, N.Y.: Springwater Center, 1986.

Palmer, W., *The Intuitive Body: Aikido as a Clairsentient Practice.* Berkeley: North Atlantic Books, 1994.

Papaseit, C., Pochon, N., and Tabony, J., "Microtubule Self-Organization Is Gravity-Dependent." *Proceedings National Academy of Science,* July 18, 2000, vol. 97, no. 15, pp. 8364–8368.

Parker, S., *Eyewitness Books: Fish.* New York: Alfred A. Knopf, 1990.

Richardson, C., et al., *Therapeutic Exercise for Spinal Segmental Stabilization in Low Back Pain.* New York: Churchill Livingstone, 1999.

Rohen, J., and Yokochi, C., *Color Atlas of Anatomy.* New York and Tokyo: Igaku-Shoin, 1983.

Rolf, I. P., *Rolfing: Reestablishing the Natural Alignment and Structural Integration of the Human Body for Vitality and Well-Being.* Rochester, Vermont: Healing Arts Press, 1989.

Staubesand, J., ed., *Sabotta: Atlas of Human Anatomy,* Vols. 1 and 2. Baltimore and Munich: Urban and Schwarzenberg, 1990.

Swimme, B., *The Hidden Heart of the Cosmos: Humanity and the New Story.* Maryknoll, N.Y.: Orbis Books, 1996.

Thelan, E., and Smith, L., *A Dynamic Systems Approach to the Development of Cognition and Action.* Cambridge: MIT Press, 1994.

Tobias, P.V., *Man, the Tottering Biped: The Evolution of His Posture, Poise and Skill.* Kensington, New South Wales, Australia: University of New South Wales, 1982.

Todd, M. E., *The Thinking Body: A Study of the Balancing Forces of Dynamic Man.* New York: Dance Horizons, 1937.

Warfel, J., *The Extremities.* Philadelphia: Lea & Febiger, 1974.

Warfel, J., *The Head, Neck, and Trunk.* Philadelphia: Lea & Febiger, 1973.

Wexo, J. B., *Prehistoric Zoobooks.* San Diego: Wildlife Education, Ltd., 1989.

Whitfield, P., *From So Simple a Beginning: The Book of Evolution.* New York: Macmillan Publishing Co., 1993.

Zimmer, C., *At Water's Edge: Fish with Fingers, Whales with Legs, and How Life Came Ashore but Then Went Back to Sea.* New York: Touchstone, 1998.

Zimmer, C., *Evolution: The Triumph of an Idea.* New York: Harper Collins, 2001.

Useful Websites:

www.resources in movement.com is the authors' website and has numerous articles related to topics discussed in this book.

www.somatics.de is the website of Robert Schleip, a German Rolfer and Feldenkrais practitioner. Schleip maintains a large collection of articles about somatics on this site.

www.kalindra.com/montreal2001.htm is the website for the 4th Interdisciplinary Congress on Low Back and Pelvic Pain and has a large number of excellent articles including those of Gracovetsky, Richardson, and Lee.

NOTES

CHAPTER 1

[1] Godard is our source for this approach. Tonic function theory posits four structures in contrast to Rolf's use of the word *structure* to mean physical structure.

[2] McHose's experiential anatomy curriculum (found in *Bodystories, A Guide to Experiential Anatomy* by Olsen, in collaboration with McHose) is a perceptual approach to considering physical structure more specifically.

[3] Even Rolf, known for manipulation of fascia, can be seen to have also developed a protocol for using structures other than physical to make lasting changes in her clients.

CHAPTER 2

[1] It is a polarity in thought only, of course, but let us look at it as a unity of opposites, what Heraclitus called *palintonic*. Jeff Maitland, a Rolfer and philosopher, offered palintonus as a way of describing what it feels and looks like to experience the joy of structural integration. (See Maitland's *Spacious Body*, p. 171.)

[2] From Ni, *I-Ching: The Book of Changes and the Unchanging Truth*, p. 276.

CHAPTER 3

[1] Discussed in James and Nora Oschman's *Readings on the Scientific Basis of Bodywork*, Vol II., p.10.

[2] Only in the last two decades have biologists begun to appreciate the complexity and intelligence of cytoskeleton. Formerly, the process of preparing a cell for the microscope had dissolved the structure within the cell and it was therefore not visible to study.

[3] French researchers, reporting in the *Proceedings of the National Academy of Science* have discovered that microtubules, which give cells their shape, do not arrange in an organized fashion if they develop in weightless space. However, if the new cells are spun in a centrifuge (given an experience of gravity) for the first thirteen minutes of development during the same weightless space flight, they do form the usual organized cytoskeleton. (See the Papaseit, Pochon, and Tabony article, "Microtubule Self-Organization Is Gravity-Dependent.")

[4] Eric Blechschmidt, a German anatomist, spent decades documenting the manner in which cells respond to pressure and tension within the developing embryo. His work shows that differentiation in cell development responds strongly to proximity and qualities of space around each cell. Biology is opportunistic to space at the cellular level. (See Blechshmidt's *The Ontogenetic Basis of Human Anatomy: A Biodynamic Approach to Development from Conception to Birth.*)

[5] See Peter Levine's *Waking the Tiger.*

[6] See Jones, *Strain and Counterstrain.*

CHAPTER 4

[1] From lecture notes of the authors from Godard's classes 1991–2000 in Philadelphia, Pa., and Holderness, N.H.

CHAPTER 5

[1] Authors' notes from class with Emilie Conrad, 1994.

[2] Protozoa are of the single-celled kingdom; metazoa are of the multi-celled kingdom. Colonies are colonial protozoa.

[3] *Inclusive attention* is a term introduced by Susan Borg in the Resonant Kinesiology trainings in Burlington, Vermont in 1986. Wendy Palmer uses the term *blended attention* in her writing; see Palmer's *The Intuitive Body.*

CHAPTER 6

[1] See Blakeslee's article in the *New York Times,* 23 January 1996, sec. C1.

[2] See Gershon's *The Second Brain: A Groundbreaking New Understanding of Nervous Disorders of the Stomach and Intestine.*

[3] See Brown's article in the *New York Times*, 23 August 2005, sec. D5.

CHAPTER 8

[1] In *Rolfing,* p. 35.

[2] In *The Spinal Engine.*

CHAPTER 9

[1] See Gracovetsky's *The Spinal Engine.*

CHAPTER 10

[1] In sitting position, we reenact a pivotal moment in evolution. Sitting up frees the hands and arms. We visit this step thinking about primates. In addition to freeing the hands to learn to use tools, which in turn may have brought about brain development, the thoracic part of the spine becomes more mobile. For discussion of evolution of brain with hand usage, see Tobias's *Man, the Tottering Biped: The Evolution of His Posture, Poise and Skill.*

[2] See Chapter 1 for this discussion.

CHAPTER 11

[1] Llinas, in *I of the Vortex,* makes the case that all animals have the capacity to use past and future to cope with the present. This, he argues, has been necessary for survival but it also takes present sensation and almost instantaneously converts it into a reality based on past experience. This translates into muscle recruitment that attempts to best affect the animal's chance of survival. This hard-wired strategy for learning movement at all levels of animal existence makes exclusive presence to "what is" almost impossible. He goes on to point out that brain development in all animals follows from the need to make movement predictable.

[2] See Packer's *Seeing Without Knowing.*

[3] See Gracovetsky's *The Spinal Engine.* Also see his article, "Analysis and Integration of Gait in Relation to Lumbo Pelvic Pain."

[4] See Frank's article "Working with Coordinative Structure, Tonic Function and Contralateral Gait," in the *Journal of Structural Integration.*

[5] See Richardson, et al., *Therapeutic Exercise for Spinal Segmental Stabilization in Low Back Pain.*

[6] Diane Lee, a Canadian physical therapist influenced by Gracovetsky, points to a model that is similar to tonic function when she describes her treatment approach. Lee describes a four-parameter model: (1) form closure, (2) force closure, (3) motor control, and (4) emotions and awareness.

[7] See Lee's paper "An Integrated Model of Joint Function and Its Clinical Application."

[8] Gracovetsky's classic book was published in 1988.

[9] See Gracovetsky's paper "Analysis and Integration of Gait in Relation to Lumbo Pelvic Pain."

AFTERWORD

[1] Bifurcation means branching in two directions. In this case we are sensing a body part that articulates in two directions. When we feel bifurcation, we are noticing an articulation, a space between surfaces of the joint, and we are feeling the flow of dividing directionality—from one to two.

INDEX

ABOUT THE AUTHORS

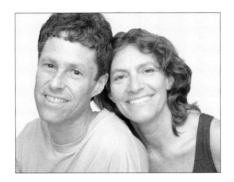

CARYN McHOSE has taught creative movement for over thirty-five years. She developed the experiential anatomy course at Middlebury College, which became the basis of *Bodystories: A Guide to Experiential Anatomy*, a book she collaborated on with Andrea Olsen.

McHose co-founded the RK training in perceptual skills for somatic practitioners in Burlington, Vermont, and uses biodynamic cranial-sacral and Somatic Experiencing® techniques in her private practice.

KEVIN FRANK is a Certified Advanced Rolfer and Rolfing® movement practitioner who also teaches Rolf Institute® and IASI CE approved courses. He assisted Toni Packer in founding the Springwater Center for Meditative Inquiry and Retreats in Springwater, New York.

Frank and McHose created and currently run Resources in Movement, a center for movement inquiry in Holderness, New Hampshire, where they live. For articles by and other information about McHose and Frank, visit the Resources in Movement website at *www.resourcesinmovement.com*.